PARADOXES OF CARE

Stanford Studies *in* Middle Eastern
and Islamic Societies *and* Cultures

PARADOXES OF CARE

Children and Global Medical Aid in Egypt

Rania Kassab Sweis

STANFORD UNIVERSITY PRESS
Stanford, California

Stanford University Press
Stanford, California

© 2021 by the Board of Trustees of the Leland Stanford Junior University. All rights reserved.

No part of this book may be reproduced or transmitted in any form or by any means, electronic or mechanical, including photocopying and recording, or in any information storage or retrieval system without the prior written permission of Stanford University Press.

Printed in the United States of America on acid-free, archival-quality paper

Library of Congress Cataloging-in-Publication Data

Names: Sweis, Rania Kassab, author.
Title: Paradoxes of care : children and global medical aid in Egypt / Rania Kassab Sweis.
Other titles: Stanford studies in Middle Eastern and Islamic societies and cultures.
Description: Stanford, California : Stanford University Press, 2021. | Series: Stanford studies in Middle Eastern and Islamic societies and cultures | Includes bibliographical references and index.
Identifiers: LCCN 2020044966 (print) | LCCN 2020044967 (ebook) | ISBN 9781503628502 (cloth) | ISBN 9781503628632 (paperback) | ISBN 9781503628649 (ebook)
Subjects: LCSH: Child health services—Egypt. | Children—Health and hygiene—Egypt. | Medical assistance—Egypt.
Classification: LCC RJ103.E3 S84 2021 (print) | LCC RJ103.E3 (ebook) | DDC 362.19892000962—dc23
LC record available at https://lccn.loc.gov/2020044966
LC ebook record available at https://lccn.loc.gov/2020044967

Cover photo: Graffiti, Cairo, Egypt. Baher Khairy | Unsplash
Cover design: Christian Fuenfhausen

Contents

Acknowledgments vii
Note on Language xi

INTRODUCTION 1

1 **SHELTERING CHILDREN** 17

2 **HEALTHCARE ON PATROL** 42

3 **(IN)VISIBLE WOUNDS** 70

4 **DO MUSLIM VILLAGE GIRLS NEED SAVING?** 93

5 **PROFESSIONAL AMBIVALENCE** 124

CONCLUSION 151

Notes 165
References 175
Index 185

Acknowledgments

I HAVE MANY PEOPLE AND INSTITUTIONS TO THANK FOR CONTRIButing to the development of this book. First and foremost, I wish to acknowledge the children and global aid workers who appear in the pages that follow. It is to them that I dedicate this book. They trusted me with their stories, spent valuable time with me, and taught me much about their lives, all with the utmost grace. In line with institutional protocols on research with human subjects, all of the names of people and organizations have been changed in this book to ensure anonymity. Although I cannot name the children and workers in this book, their kindness, hospitality, and overall generosity made the entire study possible. Through it, I hope, they will not be forgotten.

In Egypt, I benefited from the assistance of numerous colleagues and friends, including Ragui Assaad, Essam Ali, Magda Boutros, Alaa Sabeh, Adel Azer, Ghada Barsoum, Nadia Zabani, Nihal Elwan, Rana Emam, Radwa El Kady, Fatima Saeed, Amira Abd El-Khalek, Ehaab Abdou, Ahmed Zahran, Mohamed El Zanaty, Hala Hattab, Osama M. Hijji, Mahmoud Hamza, Mira Shihadeh, Oumnia Abaza, Alia Mossallam, Dina Makram-Ebeid, Nora Baraka, Sherine Hamdy, Kyriaki Papageorgiou, and Heidi Morrison. Charles Hirschkind and the late Saba Mahmood opened their Cairo home to me when I needed it and were a source of comfort and camaraderie. Saba's illustrious memory lives on. I hope she would have been proud of this work.

My passion for ethnographic research first blossomed at the University of California at Irvine. As an undergraduate there, I fell in love with cultural anthropology thanks to the friendship of Evelyn Almodovar and a dynamic group of scholars including Victoria Bernal, Leo Chavez, Bill Maurer, and Tom Boellstorff. To this day, their lessons remain ingrained in my head; they will always be role models.

At Stanford University, my greatest intellectual debts go to Sylvia Yanagisako, Liisa Malkki, James Ferguson, Matthew Kohrman, and Joel Beinin. In their own unique styles, they have shaped my thinking and writing immeasurably. I am also deeply thankful to Paulla Ebron, Miyako Inoue, Kabir Tambar, Barbara Voss, and Ramzi Salti for providing invaluable mentorship. I was also lucky to have the companionship of brilliant colleagues while at Stanford, all of whom challenged me and ultimately contributed to this work. They are Hannah Appel, Nikhil Anand, Elif Babül, Robert Samet, Ramah McKay, Kevin O'Neill, Bruce O'Neill, Brandon Wolfe-Hunnicutt, Arana Hankin, Rachel Ama Asaa Engmann, Mun Young Cho, Yoon Jung Lee, Tomas Matza, Tania Ahmad, Kristin Monroe, Sima Shakhsari, Erica Lorraine Williams, Dolly Kikon, Zhanara Nauruzbayeva, Nadia Geussous, João Felipe Goncalves, Aisha Ghani, Austin Zeiderman, Maura Finkelstein, Michael Allen, Silvana Rosenfeld, Fernando Armstrong-Fumero, Jennifer Derr, Patricia Kubala, and Dina Ramadan.

At Georgetown University's Center for Contemporary Arab Studies, I found a welcoming home among Middle East scholars as I completed a postdoctoral research and teaching fellowship. Rochelle Davis, Fida Adely, Susan Terrio, and Laurie King provided nonstop intellectual generosity to this fellow anthropologist, while Judith Tucker, Osama Abi-Mershed, Samer Shehata, Joseph Sassoon, Ted Swedenburg, Adel Iskandar, Elliot Colla, Salim Tamari, Rania Kiblawi, and Kelli Harris helped to make my time at the Center productive and so much fun. For granting me the time and space necessary to "cook" many of the ideas in this book, and for allowing me to be part of such a vibrant group of thinkers, I will remain ever grateful to the Center of Contemporary Arab Studies.

As Bates College, colleagues in the Department of Anthropology, as well as Senem Aslan, Lisa Maurizio, Áslaug Ásgeirsdóttir, Stephen Engel, and Paul Eason, helped to refine my work while making life in Lewiston, Maine, incredibly joyous, even during the blizzards. I am especially thankful for Elizabeth Eames. Her expertise in the anthropology of gender and her unstoppable social activism gave me something to aspire towards as I navigated my first year as a full-time professor. Elizabeth continues to inspire me.

My colleagues in the department of sociology and anthropology at the University of Richmond provided tremendous support as this book took shape. Others in Richmond gave valuable help as the chapters materialized. They are Erika Zimmermann Damer, Mariela Méndez, Joanna Love, Julianne Guillard, Kimberly Brown, Laz Lima, Sara Pappas, Lidia Radi, Rafael de Sa, and Elizabeth Kissling. I was fortunate to have Ladelle McWhorter as a mentor and friend. The fiercest feminist philosopher and Foucauldian scholar I know, Del has truly expanded my theoretical repertoire, making me a braver, more engaged scholar.

Numerous other scholars took the time to read and comment on various iterations of the chapters, in writing groups or at professional conferences such as the annual meeting of the American Anthropological Association, the Middle East Studies Association, and the Anthropology of Childhood and Youth Interest Group. For sharing such useful feedback with me and caring deeply about this work, I want to express my heartfelt gratitude to Aviva Sinervo, Rachael Stryker, Jennifer Adair, Farha Ghannam, Erica Bornstein, Jessica Winegar, Miriam Ticktin, Paul Amar, Omar Dewachi, Sa'ed Atshan, Faedah Totah, Andrea Wright, Diana Obeid, and Hussam Timani.

The research on which this book is based was generously funded by the Social Science Council, as well as various awards from Stanford University, Bates College, and the University of Richmond. Two anonymous reviewers commissioned by Stanford University Press improved this book by raising questions and sharing valuable suggestions. I am so grateful for the time they dedicated to making this book stronger. The remarkable contributions of the editorial team at Stanford University Press, and especially Kate Wahl, Editor-in-Chief, cannot be overstated. My deepest appreciation goes to Kate for ushering this book to completion and including it in the press's prestigious Middle Eastern and Islamic Societies and Cultures Series. It is truly an honor to be part of this series.

My life partner, Patrice D. Rankine, has given me all the love and support anyone could ask for while writing a book. For being my greatest source of encouragement each day, for remaining my greatest inspiration on everything related to social justice, and for being my person through thick and thin, I am profoundly thankful to him.

Note on Language

WHEREVER POSSIBLE IN THIS BOOK, I HAVE USED THE SYSTEM OF Arabic transliteration that is outlined in the *International Journal of Middle East Studies* (*IJMES*). However, because this is an ethnographic study conducted in Egypt, many words and phrases appear in the colloquial dialect. For example, the standard Arabic *qaf* is replaced by the usage of the *hamza* or glottal stop in spoken Egyptian. The standard or French-sounding *jim* is replaced by the hard "g" of spoken Egyptian dialect, and so on. I have transcribed colloquial words and phrases to the best of my interpretive ability. I drew on my field notes to preserve their contextual meaning. In keeping with the *IJMES*, I have omitted the use of diacritical marks in my transliterations. For English or French publications that incorporated Arabic words, I have retained the original authors' transcriptions as they appeared in the documents. Language in everyday life is fluid and ever-changing. Any shortcomings in transliterations in this book are mine and mine alone.

INTRODUCTION

LIKE OTHER PEOPLE WHO GREW UP IN THE UNITED STATES, I WAS exposed to images of suffering children in faraway lands from a very young age.[1] Television advertisements, in particular, first drew me in to this depoliticized suffering, which was, to me, clearly written on tiny, emaciated bodies, torn-up clothes, and the impoverished surroundings in which children were featured—a run-down village in Latin America or a crowded urban slum somewhere in Africa. These children were almost always captured on camera alone. Their singular, vulnerable faces gazed up at me, the viewer, as I was being hailed as a compassionate beneficiary, a savior. Through such media, and long before I began college and earned an undergraduate degree in cultural anthropology, I developed an ethic of global humanitarianism, a charitable sensibility framed around internationalism and responsibility.

At the time, I never thought of asking where these children's parents or communities were, if they even wanted the aid, or what they actually did with the aid once they received it from the organization that was doing the advertising. I never imagined these children as agents with the capacity to decide what they wanted, resist adults, or stake claims in the global aid encounter. More importantly, I never conceived of these children as criminals who could be handcuffed, imprisoned, or even killed by their local police. In fact, local governments and their histories seemed to disappear entirely from these media vignettes. Thus, watching these advertisements from the comfort of my modest yet middle-class home in the

United States, I simply felt bad for the children and wanted to help. As the popular mantra goes: doing something is better than doing nothing.

Today, many of the students I teach at the private liberal arts college where I am employed recite this mantra. A good majority of these students are majors in the global studies program, which has long remained among the most popular programs on campus. But today, in the aftermath of a once-in-a-lifetime global pandemic—the novel coronavirus—many will activate their impulse for "doing something" in the world in the United States. These students grew up as I did, in contexts where the idea of charitable giving to suffering children in the global south was abundant and framed as a responsibility of educated, middle-class citizens in the global north. In the age of COVID-19, even though media cameras (real and metaphorical) still report on suffering across the globe, they increasingly focus more on trouble at home. For instance, Johns Hopkins University's COVID-19 Dashboard tracks cases and confirmed deaths that are both "global" and in the "US." This empathy machine—the media and the conversations that drive students and others to give of themselves, locally and internationally, financially and in embodied ways—belies much of the research present in this book.

My central argument in this book is that global medical aid is a paradox of care for children and medical aid workers in Egypt. According to one definition in the *Merriam-Webster* dictionary, a paradox is "a statement that is seemingly contradictory or opposed to common sense and yet is perhaps true." In the case of humanitarian aid, paradoxes have been well-documented: humanitarian aid, while certainly well-intentioned may be neither humanitarian nor helpful in its implementation. Humanitarian aid can in fact be harmful and self-interested. Therein lies the paradox. When it comes to children and medical aid, this precarity, this paradox, is especially poignant.

I emphasize the concept of paradox throughout this book because the term most accurately captures what I witnessed and experienced while immersed in the complex world of global medical aid for children in Egypt. Paradoxes leave us in a quandary, a conundrum of which there is often no easy solution. Care, especially care for the sick and suffering child, is meant to help, ease, and assist. Care can be work, an aspect of one's chosen career or vocation, but it could also signal love, nurturance, and affection.

For the adult aid givers whose stories comprise this book, their work, their vocation, was certainly an act of care. At the same time, their work maintained or even deepened the social, economic, and political disparities that shaped children's daily lives. Medical aid comforted the immediate bodily suffering of some extremely vulnerable children, but it also prolonged the conditions that caused sickness and suffering across child populations. As a system embedded in local state structures, global medical aid did little to nothing to change the status quo for vulnerable child recipients. Paradoxically, the work of caregiving frequently had harmful effects on aid givers as well.

Paradoxes are confounding to many of us because they are ambiguous, contradictory, and often unquantifiable. Put differently, they can reflect a situation that is simultaneously beneficial and debilitating, helpful but dangerous. Each aspect of a paradox warrants our deepest consideration and attention. Paradoxes therefore require qualitative approaches to the conundrums they raise, research methods that capture the messiness of lived experience and amplify the voices of human subjects who experience them most intimately.

My findings in this book grow from in-depth, ethnographic research I conducted inside three prominent global aid organizations operating in Egypt between 2007 and 2009. However, the paradoxes illustrated in each chapter are instructive for other circumstances across the globe. Healthcare and humanitarian aid were already of great interest when I began this research, but the novel coronavirus has intensified our world's growing focus on healthcare in times of crisis. Global humanitarianism seems to direct us to care for suffering bodies, in this case, those of distant and distressed children living in poverty.[2] Throughout this book, I challenge readers to engage with the question of what we, caregivers and donors, ourselves gain from such global medical humanitarian transactions. I also urge us to consider the deleterious effects medical care can have on local healthcare workers, particularly those from underserved communities.

If empathy and charitable giving are problematic, as I will suggest, how did we get to a point where conventional views of medical humanitarian aid became so simplified? For one thing, global aid industries repackage large-scale political and economic problems, like global poverty or political violence, into manageable, individual symptoms afflicting autonomous people. This renders systemic human suffering, occurring at the macro-level of populations, solvable through attention paid to singular bodies (the micro-level) and through consumerist practices, such as quick and easy business transactions. The online donation fund for the popular Girl Up campaign is a notable example of this. With one click, I—as a person living in the global north—can donate money to girls in an African village and instantly "Be Part of Change" in a young girl's life.³ Many of my students hope to secure gainful employment within the global humanitarian industry to which Girl Up belongs. And the majority will. They make this career choice with good intentions, knowing that the industry is not perfect but that doing something to alleviate human suffering around the world is better than doing nothing while one earns a steady paycheck. These students hold on to this perception even while they spend weeks of sustained, critical study in courses on the ways in which global aid has been shown, by scholars across disciplines, to produce unintended consequences, one of which is to reinforce the global north's material and cultural domination of the global south.⁴ However these empirical realities fall to the wayside amidst the power and appeal of contemporary aid industries and what they can promise to do. Indeed, job experiences in these fields are often the springboard to advancement in our world's most powerful professional sectors, such as international law, politics, world trade, and diplomacy.

The personal and professional appeal of global aid work is particularly salient in the case of medical humanitarianism and global health, the industry that is the subject of this book. Overall, medical humanitarianism and global health are on the rise in the United States, as evident in the robust incentives directed at potential medical students every day.⁵ These messages forcefully promote international medical aid work as a way in which students can gain "unique experiences," and "bolster a medical school application."⁶ Recently, medical students were given early degrees, before passing their final exams, in order for them to enter the "front lines" of the fight against COVID-19. In such a global relationship, who, exactly, is being relieved through medical relief work? Moreover, we know far less about what medical humanitarianism does for the individual people and communities who receive it, but especially children—those perceived as the most passive and dependent, and the most in need of assistance in any society.

Global health, medical humanitarianism, and medical aid (I use these terms interchangeably throughout the book) constitute a form of global assistance that targets the biological life processes of vulnerable groups around the world. It takes, as its primary object of care and intervention, individual human biology rather than economic or political policy. As the anthropologists Peter Redfield and Erica Bornstein suggest, medical humanitarianism emphasizes the physical and psychological suffering of humans above all else.⁷ Rather than intervene on economic or political processes, medical aid attempts to alleviate human suffering through healthcare interventions and especially the use of medications.

A prominent example of this kind of work is the "medical mission," in which doctors and other healthcare workers mobilize resources and expertise and travel across borders—either for the short or long term—to voluntarily deliver biomedical care to groups suffering from poverty and/or political crisis. Medical missions are also increasingly on the rise in the United States. Their allure for healthcare workers across the global north is remarkably successful. According to the anthropologist Miriam Ticktin, the contemporary popularity of this work is due, in part, to a "new humanitarianism" that emerged in the 1980s with the work of French-based organizations such as Médecins sans frontières (MSF; Doctors without Borders). This form of humanitarianism fuses healthcare and human rights for the poor, and focuses entirely on the universal bodily integrity of suffering groups. But as Ticktin asserts, this singular focus on biology in global aid shifts action away from collective political reform, where efforts towards crafting lasting solutions to structural problems might go. Instead, medical missions and medical humanitarianism have the long-term potential to maintain the status quo for suffering groups because once the medical workers leave, the underlying problems of structural poverty and dismantled social services persist.[8] And in the case of COVID-19, those who have long suffered the most, namely, underserved and poor communities, especially African Americans, will continue to suffer after the world's cameras shift away from the pandemic.[9]

Despite the contradictions inherent in global medical missions, the overwhelmingly popular view is that they are benevolent and charitable on the part of the people doing the work.[10] This book demonstrates this in some important ways, that is, it reveals how medical aid is considered beneficial by children and aid workers. There is no question that impoverished children in so-called developing countries need life-saving antibiotics and other biomedical resources that are readily available to children elsewhere but not to them. My intention in this book is not to claim that such assistance is wholly harmful. On the contrary, I have witnessed all too frequently while conducting this research how the intervention of a healthcare worker and their use of medication immediately remedied a child's painful infection or bleeding wound. My argument rather is that a singular focus on this (obviously) benevolent side of medical aid work masks the unintended and contradictory effects it produces, consequences that we must confront if we truly care about the long-term health and welfare of vulnerable children. We must remember, for example, that the word "mission" likens global medical aid work to the colonial encounter itself, repeating a legacy whereby colonizing countries sent doctors along with religious leaders and government officials to help "save and civilize" distant non-Christian populations.[11]

Paradoxes of Care builds upon critical studies of medical humanitarianism and global health to grapple with the messy, contradictory, and real-world effects of global medical interventions with children in one place—contemporary Egypt. It asks the question of how children there receive global medical aid and then it traces what that aid does, or does not do, for them over time. My interest in these questions stem from an urgent need to hear vulnerable children's voices in the Middle East.[12] At present, a glaring paucity of Middle Eastern children's full experiences of global aid persists in social science scholarship, and even fewer accounts exist about children and global health more broadly. Instead, the aid recipients that typically appear in critical studies of global health or medical humanitarianism are adults, with little to no scholarship focusing exclusively on children, child bodies, or child-centered humanitarian policies. This gap in research is even more pronounced in Middle East Studies, which is particularly surprising, since children in the region are labeled the most vulnerable of vulnerable populations and are often the first targets of global intervention. Their bodies are routinely featured in popular media and aid policy in ways that emphasize their victimized and undeveloped status—ways that mark them as different and more vulnerable than suffering local adults. *Paradoxes of Care* provides a timely window into the human relationships, practices, and challenges attached to global medical aid for children from the perspectives of child aid recipients themselves.

The research in this book is based on over two consecutive years of ethnographic fieldwork in Cairo and an upper Egyptian village in three prominent global aid organizations based in France, the United States, and the United Kingdom. In many ways, Egypt was the ideal site for this study, because it is the Middle East and North Africa's largest and most populous country, with a growing population of children living in conditions of extreme poverty. It is one of the world's largest recipients of U.S. foreign aid and remains a vibrant global hub for international aid and development initiatives. This has been the case since the 1990s, when the Egyptian state, like others across the Middle East region, adopted new legal initiatives focused on global health and children's rights, alongside economic packages promulgated by the World Bank and International Monetary Fund.[13]

As an anthropologist intent on embedding herself in all aspects and levels of the global aid industry, I worked in the offices of these organizations as an unpaid intern in exchange for research privileges. I sat in on meetings and assisted workers as they developed policy reports, statistics, and grants for health-related aid policies. These experiences gave me rich insights into the everyday work lives of the high-ranking administrators and medical experts who produced humanitarian policies for children in the country.

Beyond aid offices, I conducted multi-sited ethnography with medical aid workers as they delivered vital care to children.[14] This movement across sites allowed me to follow workers and conduct interviews and observations in all the places where they assisted children, including a homeless children's shelter, a mobile medical clinic, a child psychiatrist's office, and a village youth center. In all of these locations, I participated in medical aid delivery myself and strove to care for children in the best ways possible. Cleaning children's wounds, teaching children healthcare practices, and completing medical logs for doctors allowed me to better grasp the intimate and embodied experiences of local aid workers. Participant observation also opened me up to children's reactions to my care, illustrating to me, firsthand, how limited that care was in addressing their conditions and the causes of their bodily wounds. The majority of the vulnerable children featured in this book fell into two main groups the aid organizations considered to be the country's "most vulnerable young," street children and out-of-school village girls.

The extended time I spent tracing medical aid encounters between street children, village girls, and medical aid workers across different sites and at different scales allowed me to understand aid outcomes beyond the conventional binaries of good/bad or failure/success. Instead, global medical aid for children appeared paradoxical, first, because it provided immediate relief for some child groups in the absence of other structures of care, mainly formal, state-funded public healthcare. In this respect, medical aid was emancipatory; it afforded vulnerable children at least a partial set of resources that they would otherwise not have. In addition, it granted them new systems of social solidarity to draw on, as well as compassionate engagements from adult healthcare workers during aid encounters.

At the same time, global medical aid had harmful effects for children. Global aid policy framed children as passive, compliant, and purely innocent sufferers. It constructed them through a model of the child based on international children's rights, whereby children are autonomous subjects yet entirely dependent on adults. While on the surface these approaches to the child may seem accurate or necessary to a concerned, middle-class population in the global north, they nonetheless eclipsed children's individual agency and decision-making capacities in places where they must be empowered, such as the streets of Cairo or an impoverished village in southern Egypt. This elision of agency in policy silences children because it renders their political and economic participation invisible, as well as their status as objects of state violence and control. It ignores the various ways in which children have been empirically studied by scholars of cross-cultural childhood as active agents in their own right. In these works, children are subjects who shape social relations and the world around them; they are meaning-makers rather than passive objects who simply absorb their circumstances devoid of power.[15]

The children I came to know intimately and on a daily basis during my time in Egypt had to assert their agency while managing extreme poverty and structural violence every day. They were caretakers as well as dependent subjects who negotiated social obligations and kinship ties alongside their vulnerable humanitarian recipient status. Poverty persisted in their lives when they were not in the care of global aid organizations. And yet, global aid policy constructed them as passive, pure sufferers and as victims who should naturally accept the resources, care, and governance adult humanitarian aid workers provided. For these children, accepting an ascribed victim status also meant an elision of their power and their own calls for collective social justice—for safety from the police and for economic equity. This was why, as the following pages will demonstrate, children often decided to reject medical aid and adult care, opting instead for independence from aid workers and a sense of control over their own bodies and lives.

Moving beyond global policy to the humanitarian encounter itself, global medical aid could be harmful for children because it often worked to govern their daily practices as it did to heal superficial wounds or prevent infections. Aid workers strove to instill new biomedically "healthy" habits into children according to global policy recommendations. This process was designed by health experts to be in the child's best interest, but many of the children I observed resisted some form of biomedical intervention, because it required a degree of docility from them that they were unwilling or unable to give. Rather than passively receive care, as policy assumed, these children attempted to reshape the humanitarian encounter itself according to their own desires and in ways that increased their power with aid workers. In turn, humanitarian doctors and other aid experts had to reshape their medical practices in order to meet children's demands. The result in humanitarian aid delivery to children was a medical encounter where power between the aid giver and receiver moved both ways, resembling what the anthropologist Jean Hunleth calls a "two-way street."[16]

Given these complex and contradictory realities, in this book I approach global medical aid for the child less as a panacea for childhood bodily suffering and more as a form of humanitarian government that attempts to craft healthy child populations through discipline and regulatory biomedical interventions. As scholars of humanitarianism have shown while drawing on the work of the late French philosopher Michel Foucault, humanitarian government attempts to manage vulnerable populations by focusing on individual biological life processes. This approach recognizes global humanitarian action as a key tactic of "government," whereby power exceeds the interventions of the state to include international nongovernmental bodies like aid organizations. Working from sites spanning sub-Saharan Africa to western Europe, these scholars contend that compassionate engagements and care work focused on the body are absolutely central to the work of humanitarian government. They have also shown how humanitarian government invariably produces hierarchies among human beings (for instance, who constitutes a worthy humanitarian subject and who does not?), since "humanity" itself within humanitarian government is in flux and increasingly conceived of as a manipulable object.[17] My approach to humanitarian government is similar to those of these scholars, but it extends their work by moving beyond the normative adult body as the key site of global medical humanitarian intervention and government practice to explore the universalized and suffering child body as an object of global care and regulation.[18]

In the context of this book, therefore, I conceive of the work of global medical aid best through the metaphor of a Band-Aid being placed, time and time again, on a deep and recurring wound.[19] Band-Aids can be helpful, but they are superficial and designed to manage the most minor of wounds. They offer temporary relief, but do not get to the heart of the problem, in this case, childhood bodily illness and suffering born from social, economic, and political disenfranchisement. In addressing biological pathologies, in attempting to manage children and produce new "healthy" child subjects, global medical aid in Egypt kept the structures that caused children's suffering intact while repositioning children as victims, and as passive objects of the aid organization's care. In other words, global medical aid remedied some individual wounds but it left the forces that produced those wounds untouched—forces that continue to shape countless children's lives in and beyond Egypt.[20]

Global medical aid for the child in Egypt is paradoxical in other ways. Each chapter of this book highlights a paradox from the perspectives of local aid workers who understood their roles as dually beneficial yet limiting, and as promising yet frustrating. The vast majority of these workers were Egyptian doctors, lawyers, child-rights activists, and other healthcare workers who were part-time employees of global aid organizations and who worked other jobs to supplement their incomes. They forged intimate relationships with children as they attempted to assist them while meeting global policy goals. These aid givers frequently renegotiated and improvised their medical practices in order to manage the unintended consequences of aid—those gaps left open between global aid policy expectations and unanticipated grounded realities.[21]

One notable consequence of global aid with children was the gendered hierarchy medical interventions intentionally or unintentionally established between children on the ground. For example, vulnerable girls were deemed by aid workers to be among the most innocent of children and therefore the most worthy of assistance, while homeless and overly active boys were deemed the most threatening of young people, and thereby the least worthy of care. In this way, there were clear-cut differences in how children were approached by workers and in policy. Workers understood these distinctions through a mixture of local cultural knowledge about gender, class, and generation and the global aid policy they received from the organization they worked for. To echo Didier Fassin, who has written extensively on the moral economy of international aid, not all bodies are equal under humanitarianism. Indeed, as I will show, the bodies of children who received medical aid in Egypt were gendered bodies, both in policy and in how aid was distributed. Workers recognized that these gendered disparities shaped how they provided care to children, and they often grappled with the discretionary power they held during aid encounters.[22]

Even when this work came with professional entitlements like paychecks and valuable experience, medical humanitarian aid work was arduous labor for these workers. They dedicated a great degree of emotional and physical labor to caring for street children and village girls, and it at times went unnoticed in formal policy. Moreover, their work often pinned them against local authorities who resisted foreign aid intervention or exacerbated children's suffering (as was the case with the police). Ramah McKay points out, in a study of global health in Mozambique, that biomedicine is always "enacted through situated practices informed at once by transnational flows of funding, materials, and knowledge, and by located [...] practices of care."[23] Similarly, these aid workers consolidated their local knowledge of culture with global biomedical expertise in an effort to achieve the best aid outcomes possible for children and themselves. In this respect, *Paradoxes of Care* offers new insights into how global medical aid shapes both the givers of aid—from low-level volunteers to paid physicians—and its receivers in creative and unforeseen ways.

EGYPT'S PLACE IN THE WORLD OF GLOBAL AID

Located in a strategic geographical zone at the interstices of Africa, Asia, and the Middle East, Egypt occupies a critical place in the world of global aid. But recently, the entire region has made headlines because of its association with human suffering. In 2018, the United Nations High Commissioner for Refugees (UNHCR) along with the United Nations Children's Fund (UNICEF) deemed the Middle East and North Africa hosts to the world's largest humanitarian crises since World War II, and that due to protracted conflict, political transition, and civil unrest in Syria, Yemen, Iraq, and Gaza, a "staggering" number of vulnerable people—nearly seventy-one million—reside in the region, and the majority of them are children.[24] Indeed, the vast size and scale of recent humanitarian crises in the Middle East and North Africa have made news headlines and colored policy reports for over a decade now, framing the region as an explosive disaster zone, a place of immense human suffering, and a salient site for compassion-driven intervention. But the discourses and images that frame the region as a site of intervention have been with us for far longer than our contemporary humanitarian crises. Like Africa, which anthropologist Liisa Malkki has researched, the Middle East has "embodied need" on a regional scale since its colonization.[25] In its modern history, Egypt was colonized first by the French in the eighteenth and nineteenth centuries, and then by the British up until the early twentieth century. Due to its rich natural resources, including the majestic yet seemingly ungovernable Nile River, and its political location as a strategic U.S. ally, Egypt has remained an object of Western technical and developmental expertise.[26] Indeed today, Egypt is among the world's largest recipients of U.S. foreign aid.

In the aftermath of 9/11, American-based global development institutions have framed Egypt as an explosive zone of crisis, mainly due to Western fears of Islamic extremism and the steady growth of its unemployed young populations, especially poor boys and young men.[27] Egypt is the Middle East and North Africa's largest and most populous country, with roughly half of its population of nearly one hundred million falling below the age of thirty. The global aid policy approaches this young population through a curious mixture of compassion and fear. Ananya Roy explains this fear as an aftereffect of 9/11, whereby the Middle East is imagined by international aid experts as a "hot spot" of violence in urgent need of remedy if the United States, and the entire global north for that matter, is to enjoy safety and security.[28] Thus Egypt's reputation in the offices of global aid organizations as a "ticking time bomb" paints its young and growing population as vulnerable and as a global political hazard. Such global aid metaphors of the young incite fear in the global north because they are economically and racially informed. These perceptions cast Egypt's masses as other—as young, Muslim, and poor—and potentially angry should their present-day demands go unnoticed.[29]

Global health policy for Egypt similarly establishes itself through these discourses of vulnerability *and* threat, positioning the bodies of vulnerable children as embodiments of the future developing nation. In this aid policy, children are constructed as the drivers of the future national economy. Their improved health, as policy reports assert, will help engender future peace.[30] Thus, global health policy for Egyptian children is framed by policy experts around ideas of national progress, where a temporal dimension to the supposed threat they represent exists. This same policy urges government bodies, donors, and concerned publics in the north to act quickly and intervene, to save these children, before their bodies grow and they become adults. The discourse incites compassion for vulnerable children in Egypt, but it also ignites fears about what is to come, both there and globally, if the health of these young populations is not prioritized. Each chapter of this book offers a critical policy analysis on an aspect of medical aid, and suggests that stereotypes about Middle Eastern or Islamic "cultures" frame key dimensions of aid discourse for Egypt. These cultural stereotypes are attached to Egyptian children and their communities, and are maintained through seemingly apolitical biomedical "facts." Such policies, I show, are designed by aid experts in the global north with powerful public and private donors in mind, including ExxonMobil and Nike. Like biomedicine itself, these policies are not "culture free."[31] They carry with them a set of assumptions about normal "healthy" childhood, as well as about the children they strive to save and their respective communities and "cultures."

Egypt's young population indeed faces a set of generationally specific dilemmas that have worked against them. They are growing up in the aftermath of nearly five decades of aggressive state and capitalist market restructuring, deemed "neoliberalism" by scholars.[32] These processes began in the 1970s with the late President Anwar Sadat's historic *Infitah al Iqtisad* (open door economic policies), which were the result of the Camp David Accords with Israel and the United States.

In subsequent years, a series of structural adjustment programs were promoted by the International Monetary Fund, World Bank, and the Egyptian state. They set into motion policies that eroded many of the economic and social safety nets the Egyptian poor and working classes relied on. These policies increased poverty levels and widened the gap between the middle classes and the poor. Then in 2004, a new set of structural adjustment reforms further struck at the heart of the Egyptian poor, substantially eliminating, among other valuable resources, food subsidies and state-funded public health-care services.

At the same time, vulnerable and poor populations witnessed an increase in state repression, authoritarianism, and police militarization, another aspect of neoliberal state restructuring that has swept through other regions of the world including Latin America and sub-Saharan Africa.[33] It is no wonder then that in 2011 and 2013, the country erupted in a series of mass protests against the government and the effects of these political-economic processes. As the world watched through live-streaming news media, millions of Egyptians took to the streets across villages and cities demanding the demise of the regime and an alleviation of poverty, unemployment, food insecurity, and intensifying police repression.

Another major consequence of neoliberal restructuring over the past five decades in Egypt was the steady proliferation of foreign aid and nongovernmental organizations that claim to operate on behalf of vulnerable poor populations—those that have suffered the most from the retreat of state-funded social services. As anthropologists of globalization assert, these organizations attempt to "do the work of the state" following its dismantling in postcolonial contexts across the Middle East, Africa, Latin America, and Asia.[34] The organizations researched in this book represent this global trend in global humanitarian governance work.[35] They are large-scale, widely recognizable organizations; and indeed, many of my peers and academic colleagues are familiar with them, if not active donors. Although these organizations were distinct in their branding and specific focus, with respect to the forms of care they provided vulnerable children, they were very similar in their corporate, transnational structures and in the policy discourses they produced about children in the Middle East and North Africa. The local workers in the Cairo-based offices of these organizations knew each other well and collaborated across various humanitarian sites to advance the same long-term aid projects across the country. Each of these organizations foregrounded street children and village girls as their primary aid recipients and approached them as bearing the burdens of the intersecting sociopolitical forces I mentioned earlier. When it came to their medical aid programs, the organizations framed biomedical care work around individual child bodies and their "right to health." They borrowed the language of international child rights and Western categories of the self and family to narrate suffering and craft their standardized policies.[36]

THE STRUCTURE OF THE BOOK

Collectively, the chapters of this book are episodic, and each features a different kind of intervention as it was experienced with a different child group. While each chapter can stand on its own, together the episodes tell a full story about the gaps that exists between global aid policy for vulnerable children and its local implementation. Beginning in a children's shelter, moving on to a mobile medical clinic, then to a child psychiatrist's office, and eventually to a village youth center, each chapter illustrates specific, paradoxical dimensions of medical aid work in practice. The final ethnographic chapter focuses exclusively on the aid workers and child-rights experts who translated international children's rights and global biomedical discourses and remade them into national policy for Egypt. Thus, by moving from the grounded particularities of medical aid with children to an examination of Egyptian expertise inside the offices of large-scale global aid organizations, this book provides a multi-scaled narrative road map for scholars and students of global aid, as well as medical practitioners, aid workers, and concerned publics who hope to make a difference in the world either by providing aid to vulnerable groups, donating resources to humanitarian causes, or becoming more attuned to how global aid sustains our world's enduring inequalities.

Overall, *Paradoxes of Care* confronts the limits of global medical aid for children in Egypt and encourages a reexamination of child-centered medical humanitarian action worldwide. The book does not attempt to offer concrete policy recommendations as to how we can do more or better global aid work for children, although readers can use the book for that purpose if they wish. Instead, the chapters provide empirically grounded answers to some of the most difficult questions plaguing our current moment of global medical relief, such as what, exactly, happens when children are the primary beneficiaries of biomedical aid? I have attempted to capture the relationships that unfold on the ground through that process and from the perspectives of all those involved—children, aid workers, and biomedical aid policy experts. As an anthropologist, I strove to do this with as much ethnographic accuracy as possible, knowing that the "truths" of anthropological knowledge are always partial and that my own subjectivity as an Arab American woman and Jordanian native shaped the data I was able to collect and interpret.[37]

No ethnographic study is pure and complete. However, it is my hope that the research I provide in the following pages serves as a springboard for deeper and more critical conversations about how children around the world struggle for a good life within the confines of their local situations. I have written the book in a style that, I hope, is accessible to the broadest readership possible yet which nonetheless still illuminates the many complexities and inconsistencies global aid engenders for individual children and aid workers. As each chapter elucidates, vulnerable children work towards their health, safety, and social justice in diverse ways, both with and without global medical assistance. They do so while making decisions for themselves and others, and as subjects who are fully embedded in the promises and perils of local and global politics. As their stories render the model of the child in international children's rights especially problematic and paradoxical, they shed light on the possibility of reimagining "help" for our most vulnerable populations.

Chapter 1

SHELTERING CHILDREN

WINTER DAYS IN CAIRO ARE REFRESHINGLY CHILLY AND BREEZY, A welcome change from the suffocating heat and humidity of summers. The wind blowing in from the Mediterranean is less powerful compared to other seasons, and the constant sun and relatively cool temperatures make it the ideal time for outdoor activities. In January 2008, during one such crisp winter afternoon, I met ten-year-old Nada for the first time. She was playing outside with other children, in the courtyard of a street-child shelter run by Children's Charity International (CCI; the name has been changed to protect anonymity), one of the most prominent global aid organizations working in Egypt. I had just begun ethnographic research at CCI and would eventually spend the majority of 2008 volunteering, observing, and interviewing children and aid workers about their experiences there. Funded by its main headquarters in Paris, CCI Cairo was highly respected among humanitarian workers and the general public. Its signature emblem, its name in red letters, was instantly recognized by many throughout Cairo. It defined itself in formal policy as a secular organization, with well-established programs in Europe and across the Middle East, including Morocco, Yemen, Lebanon, and the West Bank/Gaza. It was best known for advancing children's rights in the Middle East, while integrating innovative healthcare programs into its programs for vulnerable children.

Rather than remain inside the hollow two-story building that sat in the center of the compound, where classrooms and offices were rarely occupied, I spent most

18   SHELTERING CHILDREN

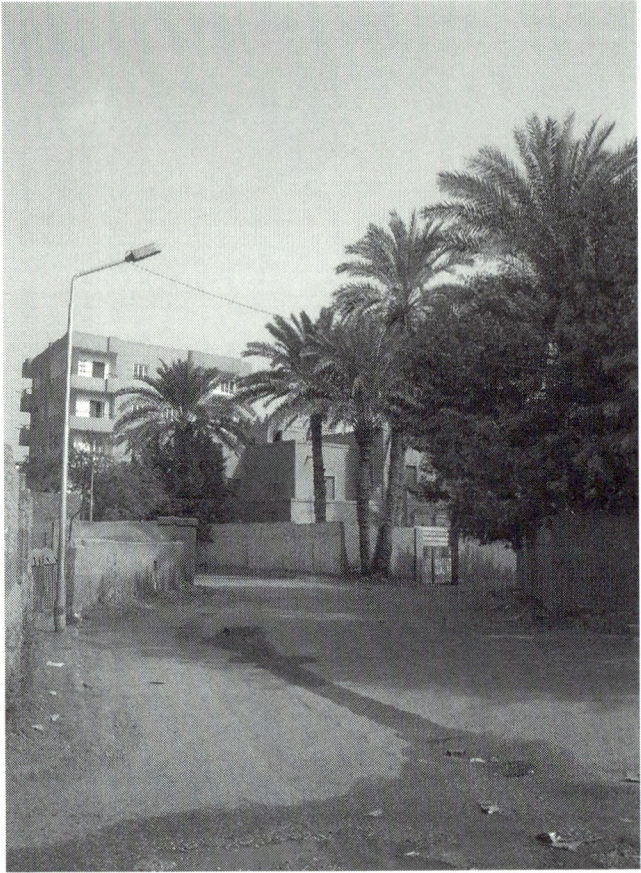

FIGURES 1 AND 2 (opposite page). The working-class neighborhood where CCI's street children's shelter is located. Cairo, 2009. Photograph by the author.

of my days at CCI's children's shelter in its spacious courtyard. That's where most of the children spent their time and where workers engaged children the most. Between thirty and forty children ate their meals in the courtyard each day on large wooden picnic tables arranged neatly, side by side. Children also exercised, played games, and received routine medical care in this courtyard under the watchful gaze of humanitarian doctors, nurses, and aid volunteers. The courtyard's wide walled enclosure gave aid workers the space necessary to organize and manage large groups of children easily. The children themselves preferred to be outside in

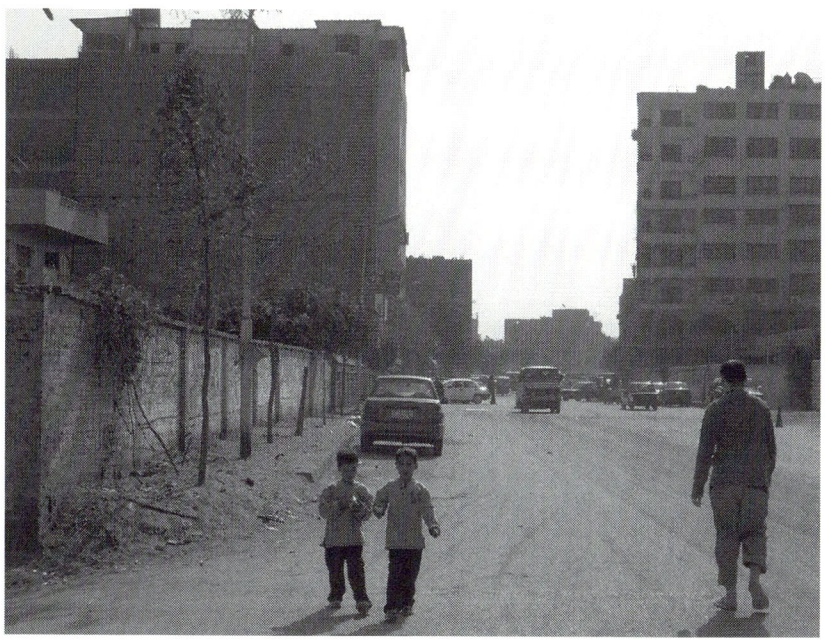

the courtyard. Sun, sand, and swaying palm trees overhead tended to ease burdensome experiences for them, such as being disciplined by an aid worker or waiting in line to receive medical attention. Nada was always at the center of action in this courtyard. Whenever children were running, screaming, or playing games, she was there, being exceptionally vocal or rambunctious. She was a talkative, gutsy girl who on the surface seemed to fall squarely within the organization's formal category of "street child"—a person under the age of eighteen who was either homeless or abandoned and therefore extremely "at risk" of suffering from illness and bodily harm. As such, she constituted the ideal child aid recipient in CCI policy. She was quickly welcomed into the shelter community by aid workers from the moment of her arrival, nearly two years before I arrived there.

The afternoon I met Nada, I was also getting to know Amira, an earnest, upbeat aid volunteer and Cairo native who was working on a master's degree in art. Amira was in her early twenties, and had over a year of experience volunteering at the shelter. When not working part-time as a graphic designer and attending classes for her degree, she spent her remaining free time volunteering at CCI. She loved children and wanted to engage in meaningful work that benefited them, which she viewed as also benefiting the broader public and Egyptian nation at large. She intimated that when children were taken off the streets, housed, and cared for in a shelter like that of CCI, it helped to create a better and more humane society, a more civil society, and it helped to improve Egypt's image among foreigners.

While we sat on one of the courtyard benches soaking up the sun and watching children play one afternoon, Amira began talking about the children around us. She described their life predicaments and detailed the specificities of their personalities. Some were quiet and obedient, she stated, while others were burdensome and difficult to oversee because of their tragic life circumstances and abrasive attitudes. As birds chirped overhead, mingling with the sounds of children playing, she began discussing the circumstances of Nada's complicated life. She felt that Nada had to creatively navigate multiple worlds and social obligations while receiving care from CCI. Amira continued to excitedly speak about Nada, "She is so outgoing and loves to talk. She is not shy at all. She loves to meet new people." But soon after suggesting that I speak with Nada, Amira warned me about her tendency to be willful and dishonest. "Be careful," Amira cautioned, "She is strong willed and sometimes lies. So don't believe everything she says to you. She is very tough [*awiya*]." In the following days, other aid workers shared similar remarks about Nada and stated that she was a "tough" and "clever" girl who was a leader to the younger children, but hard to manage. Over time, I realized that Nada had a complex relationship with aid workers at the shelter. They viewed her as having a strong-willed attitude and an ability to skillfully negotiate situations and to even "lie" to adults in order to get what she wanted, whether it be extra affection or a sugary snack during mealtime. They regarded some adults, including new foreigners and volunteers like myself, as vulnerable to Nada's manipulations and powerful charisma.

Aid workers seemed to approach Nada ambiguously, as a vulnerable and suffering street child who deserved compassion and care, but also as an active decision-maker who understood herself as an agent in the shelter. Throughout the coming months, I watched as aid workers disciplined Nada or attempted to correct her behavior by ordering her to comply. They used a stern voice and insisted she listen to them. At other times, they punished her by excluding her from games or outdoor activities with other children. Sometimes they even withheld attention from her as a tactic to get her to behave, or to express their disappointment

SHELTERING CHILDREN   21

over her tenacity. Over time, the manner in which aid workers talked about Nada and the ways in which they engaged her seemed oddly contradictory to me. CCI claimed to be a place that offered refuge and care to vulnerable street children, and yet aid workers' engagements with Nada wavered between admiration and frustration, compassion and disciplinary control.

This chapter centers on such contradictions, drawing on Nada's entanglements with aid workers at CCI. With her strong will and tenacious spirit, Nada helps illuminate a key paradox of care that lay at the heart of everyday life at this homeless children's shelter. In short, aid workers saw Nada as both vulnerable and powerful. This ambiguity produced tensions in their daily encounters, exposing larger contradictions in how global medical aid is experienced on the ground by children in spaces such as shelters, where each child's movements and bodily practices are heavily regulated by workers over long periods of time. CCI policy described the shelter as a space governed by the doctrines of international children's rights and Western biomedicine, a place where children could receive vital shelter, food, and medical care over an indefinite period of time if they were homeless or abandoned. In this policy, aid workers were tasked with an ambitious and totalizing mission: they had to oversee all of children's daily activities and their sleeping quarters, distribute food, and ensure that children showered and adhered to daily hygiene practices. Foreign and local humanitarian doctors, clinicians, and nurses visited the shelter regularly to provide medical care, performing yearly healthcare checkups and physical examinations of all children. When emergency care was necessary, they were always on hand to provide it or prescribe medication.

As the months passed since my initial discussion with Amira on the courtyard bench, I got to know Nada much better. It was striking to me how constantly she pushed the boundaries of adult authority at the shelter. Undeterred by the discipline she routinely received, she remained defiant of the adults around her, leaving irresolvable tensions between them for weeks. Conflicts between her and other children were common as well. Children frequently had crying fits when Nada asserted herself with them, such as when she claimed a coveted toy or occupied a prized space in the courtyard. In these moments, Nada displayed her power, autonomy, and independence. Aid workers were always quick to intervene by attempting to correct and control her. As months passed, it became clear to me that in exchange for living in this shelter and receiving its resources, Nada was expected to embody docility and "healthy childhood," and be a cooperative child. Yet for children like her, this was a heavy price to pay. It meant a loss of her personal agency and the inculcation of new regulatory practices that were at odds with her sense of self.

CRAFTING HEALTHY CHILDHOOD

It was relatively easy to miss CCI's street children's shelter if you drove by it in a taxi during the hustle and bustle of Cairo morning traffic, which was usually the atmosphere when I arrived to volunteer. It was located in Giza. The dusty streets of the surrounding neighborhood were always packed with honking cars and meandering pedestrians. The shelter's thick gate—sturdy and ostensibly protective of the children behind it—was splashed with colorful graffiti. It was made of neutral-toned sand-colored cement, which blended in perfectly with the semi-paved, half-sand, half-concrete streets. A four-story flat-topped building sat at the center of the gate, resembling many of the tall apartment blocks that snaked around the compound. Palm trees, tall and verdant, flanked the periphery of the shelter along with several smaller, lanky trees. Their swaying fronds, full of life, added a much-needed splash of green amidst the monotone sand and cement. In this working class residential neighborhood, the shelter was an impressive structure despite the fact that it blended, perfectly, into the sandy streets where it was nestled.

Giza is situated slightly southwest of Cairo on the banks of the Nile River. As I drove in on my taxi ride each day, inching closer to the shelter, car horns buzzed louder and flocks of pedestrians swelled, signaling our proximity to a major thoroughfare. Several blocks away from the shelter sat the world-famous Pyramids, the majestic tops of which can be seen from the shelter's sandy courtyard. The Pyramids of Giza remain one of the world's most prominent tourist destinations, and like other ancient sites in Egypt, it was a hot spot for informal child labor. Swarms of tourists, mainly from the United States, Western Europe, and the Arab Gulf states, descended upon the area year-round, providing ample opportunity for informal networks to flourish and children to earn cash.

In 2004, CCI and the Egyptian state recognized that there was an active and highly visible street-child population in and around the Pyramids. Seeking to address the "problem," they spearheaded the construction of a homeless children's shelter just a few blocks away from the tourist site. Since the 1990s, major global aid organizations labeled Cairo's growing street-child population a national problem and a moral emergency. In addition, reports considered children living on the streets a threat to public health and stark evidence of the country's failing economic and social policies. The state had a further interest in supporting this narrative because tourism is among the country's largest industries and income generators. For the state, street children were out of place and signaled economic and moral decline, they damaged Egypt's image abroad. The so-called cleansing of the area around the Pyramids would be a humanitarian effort towards children but also a move that would ostensibly strengthen foreign tourism and help quell the potential threat street children pose towards public health and safety. CCI was already active with street-child initiatives in Egypt, but with renewed state assistance it erected a full-time shelter that would serve any street child under the age of eighteen. CCI policy stated that with street children confined to one space and accessible to aid workers every day, medical interventions would be easier to administer and have a greater, lasting impact on the street-child population. In sheltering Cairo street children, CCI generated medical knowledge about them, including yearly examinations and mental health reports. This knowledge circulated through state and aid offices and reaffirmed the efficacy and successes of CCI's global aid work, helping to sustain funding for the shelter and ensure its persistence.[1]

Western biomedical healthcare and the discourse of universal "healthy childhood" permeated all aspects of life at CCI's children's shelter. Health began with nutrition. Every day, aid workers served children three balanced meals. In discussing the value of these meals, Amira emphasized the high quality of food and drinks that were distributed, all of which were funded by CCI's Paris headquarters. "Now these are really great meals, complete meals," she stressed, forming a large circle with her hands to stress the well-roundedness of the food. "Children here get the best [food]." Other shelter workers mentioned to me how substantial the food was at the shelter, stating that it was extraordinary. Mehdi, the shelter's security guard, discussed again in chapter 3, stated that children at CCI were "lucky" to have these healthy meals because in many of the households surrounding the shelter, families could not afford the same food on a daily basis. A typical breakfast, for example, included freshly baked Egyptian pita bread, boiled eggs, tomatoes, cheese, and boxed milk or juice. Aid workers also had access to either sugary black tea with mint leaves or Nescafé instant coffee.

Meals at the shelter always took place outside on the large wooden picnic tables arranged in rows under the courtyard's palm trees. This dining location kept children outdoors, where workers could efficiently supervise them as they ate or played under the comfortable shade provided by trees. Meals began at regular intervals each day, and playtime afterwards was strictly regimented, creating a shelter environment that was predictable and structured for children and workers.[2]

I usually arrived at the shelter between breakfast and lunchtime. At first, I brought snacks with me for the children as gifts, such as Nestle chocolate bars or individually packaged cookies, but Amira, attempting to remain polite one day, urged me not to because, as she explained, "they will expect you to bring more each time, and then they will fight among themselves for them." Other instances left me feeling oddly out of place. During lunches and dinners, I opted to decline meals and instead sip tea while supervising the youngest children, ensuring they finished their food. Despite the hospitality of workers, who insisted I dine with the group, I hoped, instead, that my portions would be given to someone else, and indeed they always were.

Participant-observation, for anthropologists, dictates that the researcher fully participate in a "culture" under study by doing precisely what those around her are doing "in the field site." This is so that she may truly understand the experiences of her research subjects, and eventually, it is assumed, write a better, more accurate ethnography. But in the humanitarian space of the shelter, where vulnerable children received vital resources like food and healthcare, and where local, low-level workers consumed some of the same resources, the notion of participant-observation, as established long ago by disciplinary figures like Malinowski and Mead, seemed inadequate, even unethical, to me. I tried to negotiate my structural location, as a privileged foreigner and academic grant holder, by immersing myself, as much as possible, in the volunteer work other aid workers were engaged in, but without using any of the shelter resources that became available to me as a result.

In addition to balanced nutrition as a key aspect of health, children had access to hot showers, haircuts, and basic dental hygiene at the shelter. On the first floor of the building, two large bathrooms lined the hallways, one for boys and the other for girls. Each bathroom had rows of toilets and shower stalls that, to me, resembled the facilities in a basic college undergraduate dorm. Aid workers, segregated by gender, oversaw showers early in the morning. However, if a dirty child entered the shelter at a later point of the day, he or she was required to immediately take a shower before joining other children. If needed, they were given fresh clothing, in keeping with the shelter's strict hygiene protocols. Amira supervised girls as they brushed their teeth, showered, and washed their hands collectively in the bathrooms. She watched vigilantly over sinks as girls lined up to lather and scrub their hands before thoroughly rinsing with water. She instructed girls how to brush their teeth with a toothbrush, first by using plenty of toothpaste on the brush and then by moving it around in a circular motion inside the mouth. She believed it was important to teach street children these basic hygiene practices, since many of them did not have access to running water beyond the shelter and most did not even know how to use toiletries like soap and toothpaste.

At CCI, food, shelter, daily exercise, and hygiene practices were integral aspects of a daily, protected life for these children. Western biomedical logics framed these healthcare practices. They were focused on the reduction of harmful bacteria and the killing of germs, all of which were associated, in policy, with street life and urban poverty. In order to remain at the shelter, children actively participated in routine hygiene practices to maintain cleanliness, but they also engaged in preventative healthcare and wellness activities. These practices were driven by measurable global health and development indexes that targeted public health concerns, such as body weight and infectious disease. In order to meet these global healthcare standards, children received interventions including medical checkups, lice treatments, vaccinations, and even psychiatric examinations. Children also received free emergency medical aid for minor ailments, such as infected wounds. CCI trained all of its aid workers to assist with these interventions and medical emergencies when they arose. Antiseptic cleansing fluid and basic medications such as painkillers and antibiotics were always readily available at the shelter.

Other key interventions sought to educate, uplift, and empower street children, since they were not enrolled in schools or protected in domestic spaces. The shelter had informal classes set up each day to keep children busy between meals and playtime. They focused on basic literacy in Arabic and French, arts and crafts, health and fitness, and, for older boys, electrical engineering (*kahraba*). Classes began promptly after breakfast and were taught by full-time shelter workers or well-established volunteers. Amira was fluent in both French and English, a reflection of her middle-class Cairene status. She taught an elementary French lesson each day. Most children, but particularly Nada, attended her sessions with great interest. They relished repeating new words in French loudly and confidently, often giggling at the foreign sounds as they articulated them. Boys and girls of all ages took these classes together. Enrollments were inconsistent, as instructors never knew which children would remain at the shelter or when a new child would join in. As a result, lessons remained stagnant and limited, stuck at basic, entry levels. Policy reports emphasized CCI's potential for "educating and uplifting" street children, but classes appeared mostly to manage children's time at the shelter, while introducing some creative, apprentice-like skills.

After classes, usually around 1:30 p.m., lunch was served by aid workers in the courtyard. Then children enjoyed a long period of outdoor recreation and playtime. During playtime, children self-segregated, breaking off to play with others in the same age and gender group. The older teenage boys enjoyed privileges that came with their age status, such as rights over the ping pong table and soccer ball, but they were also the ones who were most closely supervised by aid workers and were given light chores to carry out throughout the day, such as cleaning the courtyard, sweeping floors, or washing dishes alongside aid workers. Dinner was served on the same picnic tables in the courtyard and always right before sunset.

At approximately 8:00 p.m., the shelter closed its doors for the night and workers packed up, heading to their homes or to the night shift of their second jobs. This is when we usually hugged the girls goodnight and accompanied them on the streets until we knew they would be safely reunited with friends or relatives. Boys retreated to a small dormitory building that was attached to the main building in the compound. Despite needing safe accommodations, girls who were served by CCI were not housed overnight. As Amira explained it to me during my first week volunteering, this was because housing boys and girls together, overnight, in a single institution would lead to sexual deviancy or even violence against girls who were already vulnerable. The problem of sexual violence, rape, and pregnancy for street girls was something CCI and other locally run NGOs were documenting at the time of my research but unable to address in formal policy. Local and global aid organizations were working with state ministries on what they called, in policy briefings, the "problem of second-generation street children." Girls were having babies on the street, and these children posed yet another challenge for the state and aid organizations. Recognizing the scale of the problem on the ground, local NGOs were perhaps the fiercest advocates for initiatives focused exclusively on street girls and their children. But in our discussions on the subject, Amira asserted that these initiatives were difficult to achieve in Egypt through global aid organizations, and were typically abandoned without tangible follow-through. Establishing housing for street girls was difficult, she explained, because of strict moral and religious codes around sexuality. Homeless girls shoulder the burden for these sexual norms and as a result are left with less institutional support to escape street life. For global aid organizations and local workers like Amira, this gap in vital assistance constituted an unresolved aspect of global aid policy and a reminder of the ongoing gender-based violence homeless girls face in Egypt.

While CCI was not the only aid organization in Cairo that targeted street children, its shelter was unique for the interventions it conducted. It integrated Western biomedical healthcare with international children's rights initiatives. By aligning its practices and discourses with the logics of global health and rights, it strove to uphold the biological integrity and legitimacy of individual street children. At the national level, these aims reflected broader efforts to domesticate an unmapped population of children who would otherwise occupy public space, especially near a coveted tourist zone. From the perspective of global health policy, the shelter was a means to care for vulnerable street children en masse, which entailed protecting them from the violence, discrimination, and "human rights abuses" associated with homelessness. For CCI, sheltering children entailed caring for them and managing their conduct. The organization sought to regulate street children's movement, and, through educational initiatives and the inculcation of new healthy habits, refashion their relationship to their own bodies and to others. CCI policy approached local aid workers, doctors, and shelter volunteers as the powerful subjects who could achieve these aims.

HEALTH AS A RIGHT OF THE CHILD

"Health is a fundamental human right of every child," CCI's reports and policy briefings repeatedly stated. When I was working in CCI's main Cairo office, children's rights (*haquq al-tifl*) were mutually constitutive of health (*siha*) in global aid policy. At the shelter, I witnessed this fusion of rights and health as I observed the strict healthcare regimen children were required to participate in, a regimen that sought to install new hygiene habits and targeted infectious disease and promoting preventative care. These practices were described in CCI policy as critical to cultivating a healthy, dignified, and protected childhood for aid recipients, a childhood that is aligned with human rights. This, for CCI, also entailed children's emotional wellness and mental health. Since the street child was a de facto traumatized subject in CCI policy, the organization actively promoted the right to emotional wellness. Children in the shelter were required to participate in activities that would potentially boost their morale and happiness as well as their physical health. Among them were art therapy classes and fitness sessions where children were encouraged to move freely, soak up the sun, let out their feelings, and simply play. These activities, particularly that of "play," were described by CCI as essential to the construction of a healthy childhood. While CCI promoted activities associated with normative healthy childhood—such as playing—it strongly discouraged adult-like activities, such as work or independence from adults. Thus, just as CCI provided shelter, food, and healthcare for its aid recipients, it also attempted to refashion recipient subjectivity according to the universal model of the child in international children's rights.

It is pertinent here that I define the child that is central to children's rights and situate it historically and politically. International children's rights define the child as a universal, free-standing individual who is vulnerable, physiologically and emotionally immature, developing, deserving of special protection, and inferior to adults.[3] This conception of the child is rooted in the modern Western notion of childhood as a distinct life-phase. It emerged in Europe between the fifteenth and eighteenth centuries along with industrialization and bourgeois notions of family, home, privacy, and individuality. During that historical juncture, childhood (a time of protection and play) and adulthood (a phase defined by work and responsibility) became increasingly differentiated, with each sphere elaborating its own symbolic world.[4] CCI crafted its policies using many of the assumptions attached to this model of the child. Child aid recipients would, the policy assumed, "passively" receive care, such as food, medicine, and shelter, from adult workers and resemble "children" who understood their rights according to these universal frameworks.

The heady promotion of children's rights is not unique to aid organizations like CCI. I began my research in Egypt in 2008, at a time when rights-based reforms had just taken hold within the country's new Child Law (*Qanun al-Tifl al Muʿadad*). In the 1990s, a consortium of large-scale aid organizations operating in the Middle East promoted child welfare using international children's rights. The reforms these programs eventually engendered, which were written into Egyptian law up until 2008, steadily aligned local state policy with the 1989 United Nations Convention on the Rights of the Child (UNCRC). These region-wide programs were part of a larger and still ongoing "globalization of the child" process that scholars of childhood have been tracing alongside neoliberalism outside of the West.[5] In Egypt, these rights-based changes to the Child Law came slowly, as only several articles of the law were revised in the first 1996 iteration. But in 2000, CCI and similar global aid organizations pushed for, and successfully implemented, more robust revisions to the law. These revisions worked for a fuller integration of the UNCRC guidelines at the national level.

In 2008, CCI's directors and legal experts worked hard to revise three key articles of Egypt's Child Law in order to better align it with international children's rights standards. They collaborated with the National Council of Childhood and Motherhood (NCCM), the state's governing body responsible for legislating children's rights. The first was Article 112, which signaled a drastic shift in how "street children" were defined in the law. The revised article reads as follows:

> Children may not be detained, jailed or imprisoned at the same place with adults. For detention, children shall be classified on the grounds of age, sex, and type of offense. Every public servant or public commissioner detaining, jailing, or imprisoning a child with one or more adults at the same place shall be subject to a sentence of imprisonment for a period no less than three (3) months and not exceeding two (2) years, a fine no less than EGP 1,000 and not exceeding EGP 5,000, or either penalty.

In the previous law, street children were described by the legal category of "children liable to deviance" (*atfal mu'aradin lal-inhiraf*). In the revised law, they were defined by the newly created category of "children at risk," or "children exposed to danger" (*atfal mu'aradin lal-khatar*). This shift in definition was critical, as it reframed children living or working on the streets from deviant subjects to vulnerable "children." By deeming street children vulnerable rather than deviant, police could not, in theory, detain them in adult prisons. CCI aid workers understood this shift as entirely reclassifying the street child in the eyes of the state from a potentially dangerous subject, requiring punishment in the same ways adults do, to a "child" who is physically and emotionally undeveloped, dependent, and in need of adult protection instead of punishment. This redefinition of the street child in law also opened up new spaces for humanitarian intervention and rehabilitative services for street children. Now, rather than punishment, street children would require care, uplift, and protection from governing bodies.

The second was Article 31-bis, dubbed the "marriage amendment" by CCI workers. In 2000, CCI pushed for changes in the legal age of marriage, citing UN-CRC recommendations on the "best interest of the child." A section of the revised article reads as follows: "The marriage contract shall not be registered for those under eighteen (18) years of age." The legal age of marriage had previously been set at eighteen years old for boys and sixteen for girls. The revision raised the legal age of marriage for girls to match that of boys. In Egypt, this was a particularly contentious change to the law. It generated fierce opposition from local groups claiming that it was a form of Western cultural domination of Egypt and a direct attack on Islamic and traditional national family values. In keeping with international children's rights discourse, the revision aimed to eradicate early marriage, a "human rights abuse." The amendment, as CCI workers explained, targeted village communities most, where, due to rural economic disenfranchisement, marriages have historically occurred earlier for girls than in urban contexts. In chapter 4, I delve deeper into the implications of this legal revision for village girls and their families, but for the time being, suffice it to say that by making early marriage illegal, the new article criminalized parents, governors, and religious leaders who conducted marriages for girls under the age eighteen. At the same time, the amendment extended girls' legal status as "children" up to the age of eighteen, thus prolonging the life phase of childhood for them.

In Egypt, some of the most vocal opposition to this amendment came from the Muslim Brotherhood. One figure decreed that the article violated Sharia (Islamic law), which states that children mature at the age of fifteen, when they reach puberty.[6] Other opposing voices included local scholars and legal experts, who warned that the new article would unequally criminalize rural communities because in villages marriage practices are shaped by local economic and social realities. These same experts went on to assert that changing the legal marriage age for girls would not eradicate harmful marriage practices. Rather, it would simply lead villagers to engage in *urfi* marriage, a form of informal, extra-legal marriage that is conducted without a state contract. This new law might have the good intention of protecting village girls, they argued, but would paradoxically increase their vulnerability to informal practices.

The third article, Article 3, focused more explicitly on the bodily integrity and protection of children, and further delineated the boundaries between children and adults. It framed children as autonomous subjects and self-proprietors. It aimed to protect children's physical welfare by criminalizing any adult who committed "acts of child physical or sexual abuse." It reads as follows:

> This Act shall, in particular, ensure the following rights and principles:
> a. The right of the child to live and grow up in a cohesive united family, to enjoy all protective measures and to be protected against all forms of violence, tort, physical, abstract, or sexual abuse, negligence, omission, or any other forms of abuse and exploitation.

b. The right to be protected against all forms of child discrimination on grounds of place of birth, parents, gender, religion, race, hindrance, or any other condition, ensuring actual equal utility of all rights.

c. The right of children to be able to form their own viewpoints [and] to have access to such information as enables them to form and express their opinions and viewpoints, which shall be heard in all matters in connection therewith, including administrative and judicial proceedings as per the procedures and measures to be determined hereunder.

The protection of children and their best interest shall take priority in all childhood-related resolutions and procedures, irrespective of the authority that issues or undertakes such procedures.

By emphasizing children's bodily autonomy and vulnerability to violence, this revision placed greater emphasis on children's health. In asserting that children were to "be protected from all forms of violence," the new law prohibited practices that would threaten the physical well-being of children, even acts committed by family members.

When added to the legal redefinition of street children as "children at risk," the restructuring of the marriage age and this criminalization of "child abuse" served to dramatically redefine the boundaries between childhood and adulthood in Egypt, meeting UNCRC and international children's rights standards. These revisions further entrenched Western biomedical and developmental policy frameworks into local definitions of children and childhood. The child was defined in this new law as having an underdeveloped outer body and vulnerable inner emotional world. In these ways, Egypt's new Child Law redefined normative childhood in Egypt and imposed greater biomedical authority on childhood. Paradoxically, these changes increased both the individual autonomy of children and their dependency on adults.

Beyond Egypt, where similar legal transformations have taken place over child welfare, there has been friction, if not widespread resistance, to the global exportation of Western perceptions of the child through children's rights. These cases mirror many of the critiques about what human rights policies actually do in the world.[7] While the protection of individual suffering children may be their ultimate goal, children's rights have been deemed by scholars of childhood as serving the needs of the modern bureaucratic state in its effort to govern populations.[8] Moreover, international children's rights have been recognized as promoting

32   SHELTERING CHILDREN

one universal cultural model of the child, a model that reflects Western ideals and middle-class domesticity. This model has proven to be more harmful than good for children living in extreme poverty and structural violence in the global south, but also increasingly in the global north. For instance, in her research on child prostitution in Thailand, Heather Montgomery revealed the dangers inherent in implementing children's rights among a population of child sex workers who live in informal "slums," where the harsh complexities of their daily lives are completely overlooked in rights discourse on ideal childhood. Entire family livelihoods depend on the income generated by child sex workers in these areas. Eradicating sex work without attention paid to the local economic and social conditions that propelled children to engage in sex work overlooks the concrete ways in which children must survive every day. As Montgomery illustrates, children in developing countries have always worked, married, and had children younger than their Western counterparts. Rather than globalizing a Western model of childhood, the vast structural inequalities between the north and south, between middle-classes and the poor, should be exposed in child rights policy. Scholarship such as this reveals how although rights policies may be benevolent, they can also be dangerous when promoting an unchanging standard for young people, who, as Montgomery emphasized, "clearly never will have any meaningful right to this sort of childhood."[9]

Another contradiction of children's rights policy is that it constructs children as passive and depoliticized subjects who should be segregated from adults experiencing the same conditions. While, again, ultimately this is meant to protect children in a spirit of benevolence, in many instances, such as in the case of child soldiers in Africa, depoliticization strips children of their voices and agency and does little, if anything, to reverse the political conditions to which they are subjected.[10]

Similar rifts between the realities of structural violence and the ideals enshrined in international children's rights were palpable to me at CCI's shelter. Children there engaged in rights-based activities and healthcare practices that did not intervene in their poverty or alter their status as disenfranchised children who lived, worked, and actively negotiated their lives on the streets. To better demonstrate this rift, I return to my observations of Nada in and beyond the shelter to show how she challenged the model of the child enshrined in children's rights, while rejecting biomedical care as a decision-making subject.

MEDICINE, WORK, AND CHILDREN'S RESILIENCE

A few weeks into my research at the shelter, I was still getting used to daily rhythms and routines of the community: breakfast, followed by classes, then sports and recreation time, and finally dinner. One afternoon at around 3:00 p.m., as children played in the courtyard, I watched them line up to receive lice medication treatment. As a participant-observer, I was still unclear about my role with the children when it came to such mandatory medical treatments. The children were not easily managed as a group, and many of them, particularly the older boys, did not succumb to coerced interventions like the one I was about to witness. I stood at the end of the courtyard looking on, trying my best not to interfere as aid workers struggled to round up the children. Sally, a seasoned CCI aid worker who was known as the shelter's matriarch, was in charge of dispensing the lice medication. She was well respected at the shelter and often had little trouble getting children to behave or listen to her. She was the worker with the most seniority, having been hired by CCI when it opened the shelter in 2004. Usually jovial and talkative with children, she had a serious look on her face that afternoon, one that indicated to me that an important intervention was about to take place. She wore blue surgical gloves and carried a bottle of liquid medication in one hand. Amira had arranged two rows of plastic chairs in the center of the courtyard for the children to sit in. Soon after Sally stood near the chairs and signaled to Amira that she was ready, a group of boys aged ten to fifteen circled her and waited for their turn. They joked around with Sally by asserting she needed treatment too, but crinkled their noses and cringed in annoyance once the medication hit their scalps. As each boy sat, Sally's hands guided their heads to the right and then the left as she dutifully parted hair and poured medicinal liquid on scalps.

By the time several boys had received their treatments, the younger children—aware that they were next—started to scramble. Some ran into the building, others grabbed each other and jumped up and down, attempting to avoid Amira and Sally. Nada spotted me in the distance and, perhaps sensing my discomfort with the scene, dashed towards me for protection. She had a tiny body that made her look far younger than she was. Out of all the children who were visibly avoiding Sally's lice treatment, Nada was the most vocal in expressing resistance. She had a look of desperation on her face as she maneuvered behind me, wrapping her arms around my waist, and nuzzling her head into the small of my back. She stood there breathing hard for a minute, and I felt her thin body shake. Wanting to soothe her,

I reached back to softly pat her shoulder and asked her what was wrong. "I don't want it, it hurts!" she wept while hopping up and down, keeping her face firmly hidden in my back. I realized I was stuck in the difficult position of coaxing her into the treatment, although I was painfully aware of how much she dreaded it. Thoughts raced through my mind about how my position at the shelter compelled me to, first and foremost, assist aid workers in their day-to-day activities. I could therefore no longer be the anthropologist who respected children's wishes above those of adults. I felt a tinge of guilt as I encouraged Nada to receive the treatment. "Don't be afraid," I mumbled awkwardly, not knowing what else to say, "It's just medicine, don't worry . . ." (*di dawa bas, ma ti'la'ish*). But Nada simply repeated that she did not want lice medication.

Lice treatments were a mandatory monthly precautionary measure at CCI. They were dubbed in policy a compassionate intervention, meant to ensure that individual children were not contaminated, and that the shelter community remained sterile and healthy. But that afternoon I learned that lice medication was painful for the children. As Sally worked the liquid onto scalps, children sat with their closed eyes and bodies tensed. The liquid stung and lingered while it worked to eliminate living head lice and their eggs. Moreover, it had a strong, medicinal scent. Even Sally, who had administered the medication countless times, complained afterwards about feeling dizzy from the pungent fumes. During sessions when she treated several children at once, she had to walk away for a minute or two in order to avoid feeling faint and to breathe in some fresh air. Even while she suffered from the fumes and struggled with the resistant children, Sally believed in these treatments and promoted them. She described them as necessary and good for the children. For her, it was one way in which the organization maintained a clean community and showed that it cared for children. With an air of maternal authority, she administered treatment like the lice medication earnestly, and with pride written all over her face.

Amira eventually walked over to where Nada—still hiding behind me—and I were standing. Reaching past me, she gently pried Nada from my body, held her hand, and guided her over to the treatment chair where Sally was waiting. I offered a few words of encouragement as Nada was nudged away. She then sat in the chair and braved a quick yet heavy dousing of treatment. Sally's gloved hands parted section after section of her thick, brown, shoulder-length hair before pouring the liquid on. Like other children, Nada kept her eyes shut throughout the ordeal and wiggled silently in her chair until it was over. Once Sally tapped her on the shoulder to indicate treatment was over, Nada flew off the chair, ran past me, and over to the building where the other children had congregated. She yelled the entire way, waving her arms in the air and patting her head for comfort. Amira turned to me and shook her head, expressing frustration at Nada's seemingly unwarranted outburst. As if to tell me not to take it all too seriously, she mumbled, "She is just a strong-willed girl." Her tone indicated that she was used to this kind of reaction from children after unpleasant treatments.

Global aid policies assume that vulnerable children receive medical aid passively. But as Nada's experience with lice medication revealed, children do not always ask for, or desire, some forms of medical assistance even if they are framed as compassionate and enacted in their names or on their behalf. By forcibly succumbing to care that day, Nada further opened my eyes to how life at CCI's shelter consisted of a range of contradictions that wavered between care and governance, compassion and discipline. On the one hand, children received resources that were vital and valued in a context of scarcity—including food, shelter, and even adult nurturance and affection—yet on the other, they were obligated to receive bodily interventions that were uncomfortable or even painful for them. Even if they openly rejected those interventions—as was the case with the lice treatment—their voices and dissent were silenced in organizational policies. Caring, well-intentioned aid workers actualized those policies, asserting authority and dominance over children.

Amira's view of Nada as "strong-willed" girl was based on her understanding of Nada as an overly independent subject. Beyond simply being sociable, Nada was known to seek attention and assert herself in situations with adults. While this perspective of Nada was often framed in jest, in passing or as a joke, it indicated to me that Nada posed a problem for aid workers, that she pushed the boundaries of dependency expected of children. As I came to know Nada better, I witnessed how this same sense of independence played out for her beyond the shelter, serving as a source of value as she moved between the streets and her family in order to make money.

Nada openly talked to me about her life beyond the shelter. When she was not at CCI, she was working on the streets around the Pyramids. She sold glossy postcards of the Sphinx and Pyramids to tourists. Nada had a mother and sister who lived with her under a bridge near the shelter. Because these family members were not under the age of eighteen, they were unable to join the shelter community with Nada. At one point, Nada had a brother, but he had passed away under unknown circumstances. While Nada spent the majority of her days at the shelter and her nights under the bridge with her family, she returned to the streets to work when she thought it would be profitable. These were key moments during the week when tourists flooded the area, typically after the Pyramids closed for the day or as tour buses arrived and departed. When I spoke to Nada about her family, she told me her father had died years ago. But as I was sitting with Amira one morning watching children eat breakfast, I asked her about Nada's family. Amira explained that her father had left the family for another wife, thereby causing their impoverishment and eventual homelessness. Amira learned this from a drawing Nada produced during an art therapy class. It was a stick figure of a woman, whom she referred to as her father's new wife. Pointing out the discrepancies between the two stories, Amira reminded me that Nada "lied" to adults and could not be trusted. But the distrust Amira felt for Nada was tempered with compassion. She attributed her lying to the emotional trauma caused by her father's abandonment and the family's breakup.

Nada was proud of the money she earned from selling postcards, and bragged to me that on some days she did a very "good" job with profits. She shared her income with her mother and sister, who relied on whatever earnings were generated from the postcards. This was a kinship obligation that was expected of Nada and one she dutifully carried out. Moreover, Nada's age, gender, and status as homeless marked her as the ideal vulnerable subject to engage in street vending to foreign tourists, who often feel more compassion for young female street vendors.[11] Nada was therefore a key income generator in her family precisely because she was the child, an ironic reality from the perspective of children's rights.

In addition to being an active income generator in her family, Nada managed relationships with other adults in her life. Tourist sites in Egypt have become more securitized in recent years, with police regularly monitoring street vendors who work around them. Flocks of informal laborers compete for limited tourist money wherever they can, and low-level police officers take advantage of this by accepting bribes (*bakshish*) in exchange for selling privileges. Nada had to tip police officers at least one or two Egyptian pounds (approximately US$ 0.25–0.75 at the time of my research) in order to sell. However, as she complained, bribing was precarious and does not always work. When she dealt with the "good police," she was able to pay a bribe and sell her postcards. But sometimes she was kicked off the streets and entirely prohibited from selling by what she called the "bad police." They refused her bribes. When that happened, Nada returned to the shelter to pass the time, or she reunited with her mother and sister under the bridge.

One afternoon, I accompanied Nada as she left the shelter to sell postcards. It was nearing 4:00 p.m., one of the busiest afternoon hours for the area. Weaving through densely packed streets, Nada and I held hands for safety. She guided me through the traffic, which became more concentrated as we neared Abu Al Hol Street—a major thoroughfare next to the Pyramids. Passersby became aggressive as they nudged and bumped into us, and I suddenly became afraid for Nada. Her tiny body seemed vulnerable next to the adults we passed. Some were carrying large silver trays of freshly baked-bread, others had bushels of vegetables draped over their shoulders, while some were office workers chatting on cell phones while walking frantically. Having left the confines of the shelter, where adults supervised the children, I now felt responsible for Nada. However, Nada made her way through the streets with confidence, as if she knew them well. She kept reassuring me that she knew where she was going, and that I should simply follow her.

Cafés, shops, and street vendors were concentrated on Abu Al Hol Street. As we turned onto it, Nada was still walking in front of me holding my hand. She suddenly steered me towards a kiosk where a middle-aged man named Abu Mohamad sold gift cards and trinkets. "This is where I get the cards," she mentioned enthusiastically as we walked up to Abu Mohamad. She pushed her way to the front of the kiosk, bypassing a group of customers. Words were exchanged between Nada and Abu Mohamad before he passed a white plastic bag to her over the counter. In it was a stack of postcards featuring the Pyramids and Sphinx. According to Nada, she purchased the cards at the negotiated rate of one Egyptian pound each (less than US$ 0.25) and would sell each for about five. To her, this yielded a substantial profit of four Egyptian pounds (less than US$1.00).

We made our way further down the street when Nada pointed to another kiosk. She mentioned that a man named Abu Ramy ran it and that he also supplied her with postcards to sell. When I asked her why she purchased postcards from these two suppliers, Nada's response illustrated how she strategically managed business relationships with both men, and that they in turn also relied on her informal labor. One day, as Nada elaborated, Abu Ramsy noticed that Nada was a repeat customer of Abu Mohamad, and that Nada, like other street children in the area, did well in selling to tourists. He became upset with Abu Mohamad, his main competitor, and began to "pressure" Nada to purchase from him as well. Nada understood that it was important to maintain good relations with both men, as her livelihood and safety on the streets depended on it. She began to alternate purchases from the two vendors, since they offered her the same discounted rate for the postcards. Abu Mohamad and Abu Ramy engaged ==Nada as an active decision-maker and as a source of business==. Far from viewing her as entirely dependent on them, both men crafted an interdependent livelihood with her on the streets.

We continued down Abu Al Hol Street. Nada walked proudly by my side, holding my hand and swinging her little plastic bag full of postcards in the other. When the crowds swarmed passed us, she walked in front of me almost protectively, ushering me along the unpaved sidewalk with grace, narrating the hidden secrets of this major street as we passed more shops and inched closer to the ancient site. For days, back at the shelter, she talked about wanting to show me where she worked. Now that we were on her ground, and she was clearly in charge, I followed her.

We eventually approached a busy intersection that was very close to the Pyramids. Nada pointed to an area full of tourists who were strolling past a dense concentration of kiosks and shops. She mentioned that was her "spot" (*makani*), the area where she usually works. Her energy shifted to one of discomfort with my presence, and I quickly realized that if I, an adult, remained by her side it would prevent her from selling, or at least from garnering the same level of compassion and attention she would receive from tourists if she were alone. Hesitant to break away, I moved to an inconspicuous spot in intersection where I could watch Nada from a distance. Nada was now several yards away from me, deep in the crowds, and seemed focused on her goal of selling. She wasn't alone. Other children of all ages and countless adults vied for the attention of the same tourists, all working persistently to sell some item or service, even when tourists ignored them or smiled nervously and walked away.

Realizing that it was time to catch a cab and leave Nada to her work, I walked up to her to say goodbye and assured her that I would see her the next day at the shelter. "Be careful," I said with a smile, hugging her. She seemed relieved that I was leaving, but I feared for her safety, even after watching her take charge on the streets. My own head was pounding from the unrelenting, nonstop noise of traffic, car horns, pedestrians, and police whistles as we walked to Nada's *makan*, which I felt could potentially cause Nada loss of hearing over time. Meanwhile, the late afternoon sun beat down on us for hours and strong winds blew sand from the streets all around us. A layer of this sand had settled onto my clothes and in my hair, which was black from pollution and car fumes. Sitting in my cab, I could still smell the scent of car emissions mixed with fire-roasted corn on the cob, which street vendors were selling all along the streets around the Pyramids. But Nada had appeared unfazed by these sights, sounds, and scents, and their effects on her body.

Because of the early evening traffic, it would take me nearly forty-five minutes to get to my apartment. Once there, I still worried about Nada and wondered if she had sold any postcards. My first instinct was to wash my hands. As I began to lather up, a stream of black water ran down into the sink; the city had settled onto my body. I thought about the dirt on Nada's hands and wondered if she, and other street children, would develop lung complications from breathing in so much pollution over time. She was small and thin and only ten years old, but she somehow managed these urban conditions every day.

UNRAVELING GLOBAL CARE: SHELTER AS COMPASSION AND REGULATION

The next day at the shelter, Nada was beaming. I arrived to find Amira and a group of children sitting in a circle in the courtyard. Nada was at the center, discussing how she had earned five euros from two English tourists the previous evening. It was the equivalent of almost forty Egyptian pounds. After greeting the children, I stood by, listening, as Nada boasted about how unusual it was to have "such good luck" in one day of work. Some minutes later, the children dispersed, and Amira privately expressed to me her distaste for Nada's ongoing informal labor. To make matters worse, she had heard rumors that Nada had a "boyfriend" on the streets already. Her ultimate fear was that she was being sexually exploited outside the protective confines of the shelter. She hoped to get Nada off the streets permanently, but we both knew that the city lacked the institutional resources for that. I sympathized with Amira's concerns, which were rooted in her sense of care for and authority over Nada.

Nada's experiences in and outside of the shelter raise critical questions about what CCI's children's shelter does for its child aid recipients and workers. For Nada, CCI's all-encompassing shelter was a space of care and protection but only to a certain extent. It was also vastly limited in the assistance it provided, because it did not address the structural conditions that produced and maintained her poverty and constant need for money. The shelter was a regulatory space that attempted to remake her into a healthy, rights-bearing "child" who practiced good hygiene habits—in this respect she showered, washed her hands, and brushed her teeth in line with aid policy guidelines. These very same guidelines approached children like Nada as autonomous yet dependent children, as de facto passive and medically compliant subjects, ready and willing to accept care and control from adult aid workers.

And yet Nada's outright resistance to the lice medication treatment she received painted a different story about how local children understand and receive global medical aid. Fearful of the medicine, Nada attempted to assert her own power during the medical aid encounter by running away and even hiding from treatment. Although this resistance ultimately failed for Nada—she and the other children had to succumb to treatment if they wanted to remain at the shelter— it was especially telling of how both children and aid workers struggle during medical aid encounters and how certain forms of "compassionate" intervention are contested and even rejected by child aid recipients on the ground. CCI policy recognized the power of adult aid workers over street children in these aid encounters, but it did not consider the reverse to be true. That is, it neither recognized nor recommended concrete solutions for children who asserted their independence and practiced noncompliance during global medical aid exchanges.

This same policy also described Nada as a "homeless" or "abandoned" child, one of millions who remain "at risk" across the global south today. Indeed, Nada was at risk of danger, violence, and exploitation on the streets. But she was also part of a kinship network that consisted of a mother and sister who, unlike her, were adults and therefore unable to receive the kind of assistance CCI provided children. The broader condition of urban poverty in which Nada and her small family lived fell beyond CCI's governing policies. For this reason, CCI's humanitarianism, its effects as an organization promoting medical aid and global health, was paradoxical for Nada while she navigated the worlds of healthy childhood (in the shelter) and adult labor (on urban streets).

By documenting segments of Nada's life in and outside of CCI's shelter, this chapter has illustrated a set of lived paradoxes associated with global medical aid for children. Nada's independence and reputation as a powerful, strong-willed girl unsettled many humanitarian representations of the child in global aid policy, and this had consequences for her in daily life. Almost immediately after joining the shelter community, I learned that Amira viewed Nada as a problem. To mitigate this, Amira and other aid workers improvised their caregiving practices with Nada in order to manage her while meeting formal organizational goals. While we often view such goals as benevolent and compassionate, even necessary according to global health and child rights logics, they nonetheless governed children by promoting individual discipline and childhood passivity. Left out of CCI's organizational goals, but no less crucial, were Nada's economic and social obligations beyond the shelter, and her status as a subject with complex desires attached to family, street vendors, and the police.

Paradoxes such as these were not exclusive to Nada nor to CCI's shelter. In the following chapter, I further document CCI's work with street children, but from inside its mobile medical clinic, where healthcare workers and children on the streets also grappled with the limitations and contradictions inherent in global medical aid for children.

Chapter 2

HEALTHCARE ON PATROL

DR. MOHAMAD WAS A PAID HUMANITARIAN DOCTOR WHO WORKED in a mobile medical clinic operated by CCI. As an extension of CCI's shelter, the clinic targeted children living and working on the streets, and was designed for those who were not able to procure regular care at the organization's Giza shelter. As Dr. Mohamad explained it to me, it was an "arm" of the street children's shelter and a critical way in which CCI was able to expand its reach to children across Cairo. By providing free biomedical care to all street children in a mobile clinical setting, CCI hoped to increase successful global health outcomes and better manage the city's visible yet transitory street child population.

One night in August 2009, Dr. Mohamad, a crew of aid workers, and I patrolled downtown Cairo in the mobile clinic. We eventually parked at a crowded intersection. As is the case with most August nights, the air was heavy with heat and humidity. Children lingered on street corners in groups at this intersection, chatting with friends and unaccompanied by adults. Dr. Mohamad began his shift with great enthusiasm, serving the children who approached the clinic. Young Ayman was among the first patients to see Dr. Mohamad that night. He entered the van apprehensively. A large, un-bandaged wound was fully exposed on his forehead, and I instantly sensed he was self-conscious about it. Eventually, he settled onto the examination table positioned in the center of the van and spoke to Dr. Mohamad candidly about his troublesome wound. Ayman had bright green eyes that provided a striking contrast to the brown dirt that covered his face. He was wearing worn-out jeans, a torn T-shirt, and flip-flops that were tattered around the edges. He dangled those flip-flops playfully from his feet as he sat on the examination table speaking to Dr. Mohamad. He told us he was eight years old.

During Ayman's clinic visit, we learned that the wound on his forehead was a result of a fight he had had with another street boy. When the wound kept bleeding after the altercation, he had paid forty Egyptian pounds (approximately US$7.25) to have stitches put in incorrectly at a community pharmacy—a hefty price for anyone living in Cairo.[1] Now the raised and blistering wound was infected and twice its original size. Dr. Mohamad quickly cleansed and sutured the wound as Ayman sat quietly, barely moving through the procedure. As he pulled surgical string through the wound, Dr. Mohamad told Ayman how dangerous the mistake he had made was, and that pharmacists were not legitimate healthcare providers in the way the mobile clinic was. He urged Ayman to never get stitches at a pharmacy again, saying, "Next time, don't go to a pharmacy. Come back to see me, OK?" Ayman appeared to comply, politely, yet dashed out of the clinic the moment he was able to. Once he left the clinic, I asked Dr. Mohamad for his thoughts as to why children would pay so much money for faulty stitches in a pharmacy when healthcare was technically free in public hospitals. "Time. And discrimination," he explained as he tidied up the examination table for the next patient. "These boys are treated very badly by our society. The hospitals are crowded and the wait time is long. There are too many formalities and lots of paperwork. In the pharmacies, they are not seen. They go in and out. No papers, no law. The kids feel more comfortable [. . .] and safe."

As this explanation makes clear, Ayman's "mistake" was actually a rational response to an urban landscape that was hostile to street children like him. Ayman had attempted to take care of his own wound quickly and efficiently, first by bypassing formal state institutions, in this case public hospitals, and next by seeking relief from a community pharmacy. Rather than encounter the state's bureaucratic apparatus, "the paperwork" or the "law" described in Dr. Mohamad's account, and confront public discrimination, he chose to pay more money for care in a private setting. By bypassing such forms of violence—state bureaucracy and public discrimination—and by seeking care elsewhere, Ayman was active in his own healthcare management. When the pharmacy stitches eventually proved faulty and the wound grew more painful, Ayman sought as-

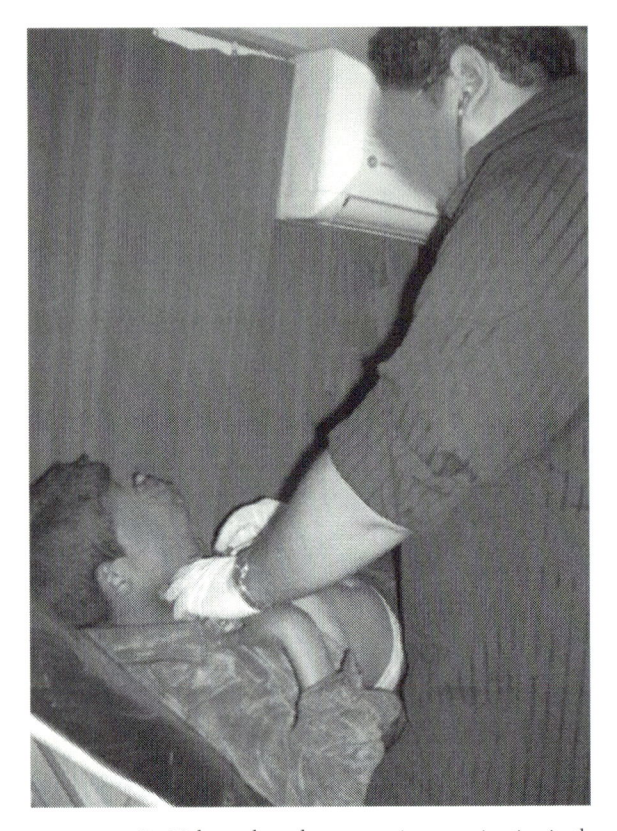

FIGURE 3. Dr. Mohamad conducts a routine examination in the mobile clinic. Shubra al-Khayma, Cairo, 2009. Photograph by the author.

sistance from an international humanitarian organization, CCI's mobile clinic. Here, CCI filled the gaps left open by Cairo's deteriorating public healthcare sector, and for a child managing life on the streets outside of protective domestic spaces. But we were unsure whether Ayman would ever return to the mobile clinic for follow up-care. As Dr. Mohamad ushered in the next child, I asked if he thought Ayman would return to the mobile clinic as he advised. His response indicated just how indeterminate mobile medical aid was with respect to long-term care for street children: "Maybe. Maybe not." He shrugged with a hint of resignation. "I never know. These kids are used to taking care of themselves. We'll see."

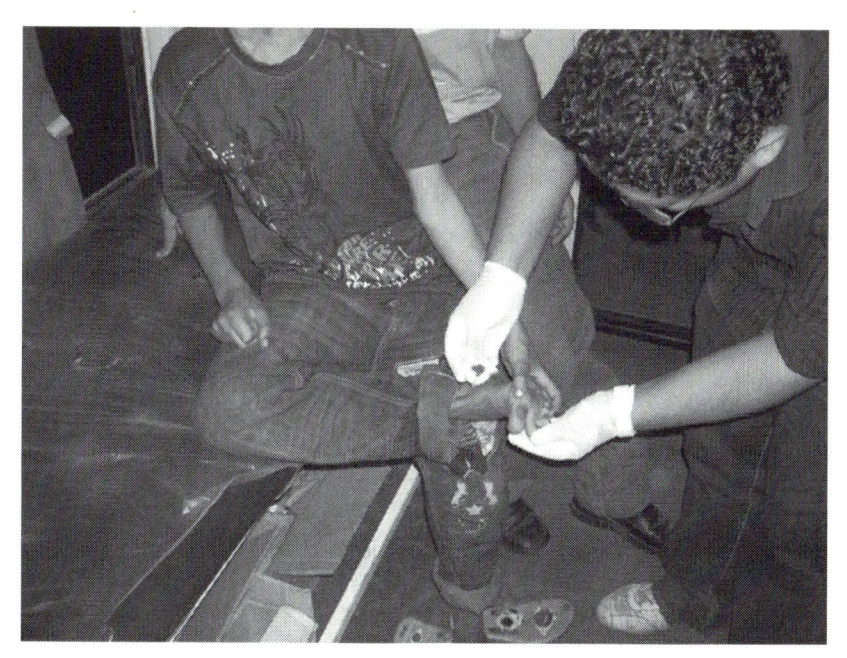

FIGURE 4. Dr. Mohamad removes a nail from a young boy's foot in the mobile clinic. Muhandasin, Cairo, 2009. Photograph by the author.

Dr. Mohamad seemed to recognize the limits of mobile medical aid with street children in this clinic. As an organization, CCI strove to provide emergency medical aid to street children all around the world, seeing such care as compassionate action and defining it in policy as a universal right of the child. Yet in practice, Dr. Mohamad struggled with an irreconcilable tension, a paradox, that was inherent in mobile aid for street children. The clinic, as he saw it, provided immediate yet limited assistance. Mobile care was necessary and potentially life-saving for countless children suffering from painful wounds and infections, just as Ayman was, yet it left the sources of street children's recurring bodily suffering intact. Ayman's case pointed to some of the underlying sources of children's suffering on the streets. It illustrated how street children were bound to real-world political conditions that rendered their use of global aid institutions necessary yet capricious and unpredictable. In having to navigate Cairo's public and private urban terrains, and in remaining excluded from public healthcare structures, street boys like Ayman strategically drew upon a multiplicity of healthcare resources that were available to them at any given time.[2] Sometimes their decisions hinged on their attempts to remain safe from bodily violence and in others, they were driven by a desire to resist the state and avoid the formal "law." Ayman chose solutions along these lines, in a manner that maximized his distance from the state and ensured a more swift and efficient healthcare outcome for him. Rather than enter a public hospital, which was, in theory, free, he sought quicker care in a pharmacy that required more funds.

It was only when the pharmacy stitches proved faulty however that Ayman turned to CCI's mobile clinic. Dr. Mohamad hoped he would see Ayman again for a follow-up visit, when he would gauge the status of the forehead wound and ensure that the stitches had been successful. But because Ayman's future actions were uncertain, as a transient street child, the progress of his stitches might remain a mystery for Dr. Mohamad. This was a space of indeterminacy resulting from mobile care. During my time in the clinic, I watched Dr. Mohamad and other clinic workers carefully negotiate this space while providing care to children as best as they could.

In charting the ways in which street children in Cairo used CCI's mobile clinic, this chapter traces another key paradox attached to global medical aid for children in Egypt: the contradictions and ambiguities between mobile medical aid's successes and failures, and promises and limitations with street children. The empirical examples about mobile medicine captured in this chapter stem from my time participating in care and observing Dr. Mohamad and his crew on nightly rounds in CCI's mobile clinic. Most of the data were collected in the summer of 2009, when, due to the summer heat, Cairo nightlife continued well into the early morning hours and children were openly working on the streets. Each night at around 8:00 p.m., after CCI's shelter closed its iron gates, the mobile clinic, with a crew of several aid workers in tow, departed Giza for one of several key stops across the city. These stops were vibrant hubs where street children could be spotted selling napkins, shining shoes, wiping car windows, or begging for cash. Work in the mobile clinic typically lasted until 3:00 to 4:00 a.m., or until the last child aid recipient received service. CCI's humanitarian reach with street children expanded considerably due to the mobile clinic. Although it was an extension of the street-child shelter described in the previous chapter, the mobile clinic represented a distinct form of intervention with street children. It brought global medical aid to them, on the streets, and operated with its own political rationalities. It generated medical aid outcomes and social effects for children and workers that differed in significant ways from those I observed at the shelter.[3]

The first part of the chapter traces the rise of mobile medical aid at CCI and examines, through its formal policies, the pedagogical dimensions of mobile care with street children in Cairo. CCI promoted an international medical-social approach to care, one in which humanitarian doctors like Mohamad were trained. With a focus on how to properly care for street-child bodies, drawing on the logics of international children's rights, this approach to biomedicine defined street children as exceptionally vulnerable and emotionally traumatized subjects. This was the discourse that guided the compassionate work enacted in the clinic.

Next, I describe aid encounters in real time, as they took place in the mobile medical clinic between children, aid workers, and Dr. Mohamad. While I observed numerous interactions during my time observing workers in the clinic, I will detail three distinct cases in the pages that follow because they demonstrated how children and other vulnerable populations in the city used the clinic in ways the organization had not intended. While observing these encounters, I quickly learned that homeless boys sought care from the clinic more frequently than any other child group, and in doing so, they routinely challenged the idea that children were naturally dependent on adults or biomedical practitioners, or that they experienced pain in universalized ways. Aid recipients sought care from CCI, but they also practiced their own healthcare management and resisted aid workers; these practices were beneficial because they often helped recipients maintain independence, power, and status on the streets. Their usage or rejection of mobile medical aid sheds light on how, in Cairo, the young male body—more specifically, the street child's male body—is a social product elaborated by specific economic, social, political, and cultural forces.[4] These young, male mobile clinic patients push us to reconsider the primary focus of global aid for children, from an emphasis on individual bodily care to a critique of the social expectations and political constrains that govern boys and young men on urban streets.

To this end, I find the medical anthropologist Arthur Kleinman's concept of "illness narratives" particularly useful in describing stories of street-child bodily injury. Illness narratives tell us about how life problems are created, controlled, and made meaningful.[5] Illness for Kleinman is always an experience that is culturally shaped beyond the body and constituted in specific political contexts. As I witnessed the life narratives of young clinic patients, I came to recognize precisely how their embodied pain was intricately linked to social inequities in Cairo. Whether they had a wound or an illness, patients approached their bodies in relation to forces beyond it, and as connected to other bodies on the streets. To mitigate the daily violence of homelessness and informal labor, these aid recipients adopted creative modes of self-care that established themselves as political actors and decision-makers. Like the children living in CCI's shelter, these patients challenged the model of the passive, dependent child that figures so prominently in international children's rights and global medical aid policy. Their gendered practices and individual experiences expose significant ruptures within mobile medical aid for street children.

THE GLOBAL LOGICS OF MOBILE MEDICAL AID FOR STREET CHILDREN

Ethnographic studies of mobile aid have begun to proliferate in humanitarian studies, as mobility becomes more central to the practices of large-scale humanitarian organizations. Mobile interventions—into war or poverty zones—raise new theoretical and practical questions about how humanitarian encounters unfold on the ground. Anthropologists have recently taken note of the various differences between mobile aid and more sustained, long-term humanitarian structures, such as camps. Still, ethnographic evidence of mobile aid as experience is sparse. One key study, however, is offered by Peter Redfield. In an ethnographic account of Médecins Sans Frontières (MSF), Redfield notes that mobile medicine emerged in a context of extreme violence. It first gained importance as a military strategy in Europe after the Second World War. Large-scale military bombing caused so much devastation that the International Committee of the Red Cross (ICRC) faced new technical problems, and mass civilian casualties. With formal healthcare structures destroyed, new and diverse methods to send medical relief quickly emerged. This innovation born of necessity marked a critical turning point in the politics of global humanitarian aid. Mobile medicine as a response to war proliferated in the following decades, but it also flourished as a means of providing basic preventative healthcare to devastated populations in zones of poverty.[6] Redfield argues however that mobile aid hardly represents a general panacea for all human suffering. In other words, in Redfield's view mobile intervention has its limits, even if it has, "long stood as a vital principle of emergency care."[7]

Today, global humanitarian organizations working across the Middle East have adopted mobile methods in order to help manage crises and get life-saving emergency care to vulnerable populations quickly. Wars in Gaza, Lebanon, Syria, and Iraq signaled a need for more expansive, continuous humanitarian support, while in countries undergoing economic crisis, such as Egypt, mobile medical aid attempted to fill in the gaps left open by failing public healthcare structures.

By the early 2000s, CCI launched mobile clinics internationally to address gaps in its humanitarian work, especially with street children who were viewed as, essentially, mobile children—constantly moving around through urban centers in search for work or safety. Echoing the discourse of other global international organizations that adopted mobile care, CCI framed its inaugural mobile clinics as necessary pioneering projects. They were characterized as an integrated humanitarian project with the power to reach all those who were most in need, even the most transient and elusive aid recipients, like street children and child refugees. These logics gave CCI's mobile projects popularity among international donors and were attractive to aid experts at local and global levels.[8] When I entered CCI's main offices in Cairo in 2007, aid workers there praised their mobile clinic as an innovative, forward-thinking intervention. During one of my first interviews, a key administrator mentioned how the mobile clinic allowed the organization to "reach" more street children than the shelter could ever accommodate. Speaking about street children, he proudly stated that through the mobile clinic, "If they can't come to us, we'll go out to them."

The mobile clinic itself was a large, white van that sported the organization's logo in bold red letters on each side—making its status as a medical aid provider clearly visible to all at night. Its sliding doors exposed a neat beige interior, resembling a typical tour bus. Two rows of comfortable seats were in the front and the medical treatment area was at the back. A thin wall separated these two interior realms and granted patients privacy during medical examinations. The back, where care took place, resembled a mini emergency room. One side housed an examination bed that was covered in plastic, while the other held a medicine cabinet that overflowed with medication, gauze packets, and surgical supplies. On the floor to one side were heaps of small black medical "gift bags" containing hygiene and sanitation products that workers distributed to street children. There were two kinds of bags, one for girls and another for boys.

Samir was CCI's mobile clinic driver and a man in his late forties. He helped distribute the bags during nighttime patrols while Dr. Mohamad treated patients. One night, he pulled the contents of one "boy bag" out to show me what was inside. I glanced at a small bar of Ivory soap, eight tiny packets of Pantene shampoo, a black hair comb, a packet of tissues, a toothbrush, and a small tube of toothpaste. He then demonstrated how pulling tight the strings on each side of the bag transformed the bag into a backpack. "This way kids can carry this bag on the streets with no problem," he claimed. Samir emphasized, with this demonstration, how the organization considered street children's mobility in designing the bags. Minutes later he opened a "girl bag" to show me that it held many of the same products, but with the addition of an Always maxi pad package. Samir asserted these products helped street children remain "clean." He hoped that when the products ran out, children would seek the mobile clinic again and ask for more. The goal, as he explained it, was to encourage recipients to return to the mobile clinic for continuous care.

Much like its shelter, therefore, the larger aims of CCI's mobile clinic were twofold: first to provide emergency biomedical care to street children who needed it, and next to inculcate, through pedagogy and gift exchanges, a set of new health and hygiene habits, thereby creating a newly medicalized and healthy street-child population. Gift bags were the main resource distributed during mobile clinic patrols, but the clinic also delivered food, toys, and coloring books to children in order to introduce play into their lives and reinforce normative childhood while they sought medical care. The resources exchanged through the clinic established relations of reciprocity between workers and child recipients.[9] Aid workers hoped to see children return to the clinic, play, and remain safe, rather than work on the streets and face multiple social dangers. Many children did just this. They greeted workers with affection upon seeing them. Workers often spoke to me about the many individual children they had known for years.

Once the mobile clinic parked in a designated spot, workers gathered children into groups and delivered speeches in an effort to further influence their practices and promote a normative international model of childhood. These informal speeches covered topics such as the dangers of smoking, stealing, and sex; and they sought to teach children how to disengage in violence and criminality, to always "do the right thing." Talks took place on curbsides, grassy patches near streets, in parks, or in alleyways near areas where the clinic was parked. Aid workers took these lectures seriously, even if they were sometimes sparsely attended or simply a way to pass the time during long nights of clinic work. We had little evidence that children actually changed their daily practices because of these pedagogical lectures. For instance, when it came to smoking—a frequent subject of the casual curb-side lectures—Dr. Mohamad admitted that the practice was still very common among street boys, and that he hadn't witnessed its decline since he began mobile aid work. In Cairo, smoking signifies masculine toughness, and street boys and young men openly smoked around us in the clinic. Ironically, and realizing the importance of smoking to manhood, aid workers even occasionally offered cigarettes to older street boys before lighting up themselves. → perpetuating cycle of social stigma.

Despite these apparent failures of aid, Dr. Mohamad and clinic workers saw themselves as conducting medical outreach through the mobile clinic and as "hailing" young people on the streets to be particular kinds of child subjects, as CCI policy dictated.[10] Along with biomedical care, education and gift-giving were important aspects of their mobile work. Like all of CCI's interventions, they were designed to care for and transform children, according to a model of childhood that was represented in international children's rights. The educational lessons assumed both a childhood dependency on adults and passivity during aid encounters, yet focused on child self-regulation and the promotion of a moral, disciplined, middle-class child self. This was most evident in mobile aid encounters that promoted play and innocence among street children, as opposed to labor. Moreover, lectures discouraged sex and smoking and encouraged hygiene, thus reinforcing the notions of purity and innocence as enshrined in children's rights. Clinic workers conducted this outreach work diligently over time, in the same areas of the city, with the ultimate goal of building long-lasting relationships with children. They believed that street children were transient subjects and that repeated face-to-face encounters would build trust and stability in their lives, ultimately rendering their aid efforts more efficacious and longer-lasting.

Filled with an array of globally recognized consumer products, from Ivory soap to Pantene shampoo, the mobile clinic gift bag embodied CCI's efforts to establish itself as a powerful authority figure for street children in Cairo. Through it, the organization sought to cultivate self-regulating and hygienic street children.[11] While I often wondered how street children would use the products they received in their gift bags if most did not have regular access to running water, I nonetheless witnessed the lasting force these gift bags produced for children. Children coveted their bags, along with the snacks and games they received from workers through the mobile clinic. Thus, while it represented a global and limited form of biomedical assistance, CCI's mobile clinic modified the local environment in which it worked.[12] It did so according to global biomedical and children's rights "scripts," allowing CCI to operate forms of childhood governance beyond its shelter walls, well into an extended landscape of need.[13]

REDEFINING CHILDREN'S PAIN: A MEDICAL SOCIAL APPROACH

In a medical training manual originally published in French and later translated into Arabic by Cairo-based aid administrators, CCI's Paris headquarters laid out a new approach to medical aid for humanitarian doctors and healthcare volunteers in Egypt. It labeled this new set of practices a "medical-social" approach to caring for the street child. The manual offered a step-by-step framework for providing superior care to street children in medical humanitarian spaces, such as a mobile clinic, specifying new scripts for speaking with and listening to street children. The uniqueness of this approach was its focus on balancing bodily and emotional care for street children. It delineated how doctors should treat children's "bodily health" (*siha*) without producing further "mental pain" (*alam nafsi*), thereby framing the biomedical humanitarian encounter as a source of emotional distress for children living or working on the streets. The opening pages of the manual describe this relationship in detail, marking a critical moment in CCI policy when children's trauma constituted the grounds for advancing better, more innovative global medical aid practices. "Emotional illness is a negative result of physical harm, such as cutting or injecting oneself," it asserts. "Pain needs to be treated, as pain that is not treated causes worry, depression, lack of rest and intense exhaustion. Untreated pain causes sleeping and eating problems, and causes children to behave more childishly. A child's emotions have a direct relationship with the degree of their physical pain."

Further on, the manual delves into the status of street children's inner worlds, differentiating between the emotional health of street children and that of other children. Here, street children were described as "unstable" subjects, as experiencing pain abnormally, more intensely. Other children, by contrast, were described as peaceful, tranquil, and rested. The manual describes all children as individuals who naturally lack the skills required to manage their own pain:

> The child that has instability in life feels pain more intensely than the tranquil child who feels at rest. [...] Coping with wounds and pain is not a skill the child is born with. People responsible for caring for children ought to develop the ability to help the child live and cope with their inescapable pain. Children who are exposed and vulnerable to street life have different experiences of pain. For instance, in many cases they may harm themselves, but this doesn't mean they do not feel pain. [...] Pain is an individualistic thing, and everyone experiences it differently.

CCI doctors, nurses, and healthcare volunteers attended training sessions held at CCI's shelter by organizational directors in order to learn this new medical knowledge. The training sessions were meant to supplant their existing habits, which the organization viewed as inadequate and unaligned with the standards of international children's rights. By alerting local doctors to street children's universal experiences on the streets, and by detailing how such experiences shaped children's inner worlds and outward expressions of pain, the manual sought to naturalize street children as emotional sufferers. As such, more compassionate engagements between doctors and street children during the medical humanitarian encounter were required to expand the organization's recipient base. The experts who instructed these classes were foreign visitors from affiliated medical humanitarian organizations, including MSF and Médecins du Monde (MDM). By training local CCI workers in these logics of care, they reinforced CCI's strong integration of international children's rights doctrines with biomedical aid policies.

The association between rights and biomedicine has garnered much attention in medical anthropology in previous years, but it has mostly emerged in studies implicitly focused on adult subjects. For instance, Deborah Gordon has carefully unearthed a historical relationship between individual human rights and biomedical theory and practice. In a classic essay titled "Tenacious Assumptions in Western Biomedicine," Gordon explores how biomedical theory, grounded in Cartesian logic and Western philosophical traditions, is inherently focused on the figure of the "autonomous individual," the basis of modern identity and claims to human rights.[14] CCI's training manual reflected a similar radical individuation of the subject, but in its case, the subjects in question were children. Its pages described its "medical-social approach" to care as a more humane and rights-friendly medical approach. CCI strove to advance the approach in the mobile clinic in particular, because it recognized children living on the streets, as opposed to the shelter, as extremely vulnerable, exposed to violence, and most in need of compassionate, rights-based medical assistance.

For CCI, street children were a child population that was exposed to physical pain, therefore its rights-based medical approach centered on the reduction of pain (inner and outer) as a key aim during treatment. CCI's training manual directed doctors on how to secure lighting and manage sounds in a clinical setting in order to alleviate street children's "trauma." It also encouraged practitioners to respect children's need for privacy and their sense of individuality during encounters because, due to street violence, street children were inherently "fearful" subjects. The manual dedicated much ink to the subject of drug abuse among street children. In an attempt to decriminalize street children for doctors, and in furthering its rights-based logics, it explained that drug use among street children was "rational," stating that children turned to drugs as a natural remedy for their pain. : "Taking drugs is one of the tools these children use to reduce feelings of pain and various other stress factors encountered on the streets," the manual asserted, drawing on CCI's discourse of compassion.

Aside from identifying drug use as a rational practice resulting from street life, this approach suggests that social conditions cause children's inner pain. The discourse individualizes pain by relegating it to the child's inner world, but at the same time it attaches pain to "stress factors encountered on the streets." In this way, CCI advanced a "medical-social" approach to humanitarian care. The descriptions above draw clear boundaries between children's inner and outer worlds, as well as children and the social world, but they also strengthen boundaries between children and adult aid workers. In the manual, aid workers are described as powerful figures guiding the humanitarian encounter. Children, by contrast, are depicted as vulnerable and pathologized, as unstable, fearful, and violated. The manual's key recommendations therefore depict the child as passive and the aid worker as active:

> a. The place: conduct treatment in a place that is respectful of a child's privacy, far away from other children. [. . .] The child will be more relaxed.
>
> b. Give the child some power or control over the treatment process. [. . .] If given options the child will feel pain less intensely than the child who has no power at all.
>
> c. Help children raise questions and express their emotions.
>
> d. Playtime: behave playfully with the child, be humorous, children will feel relaxed and forget their worries.
>
> e. Relaxation: speak to the child in a calm, relaxed voice to ease their fears, as some children are afraid of adults and physical intervention due to past negative experiences. You must not touch the child randomly or directly in these cases, as a child who has been violated would not feel comfortable.

Similar knowledge about street children was promoted in another CCI training manual. With a focus on the reduction of street children's emotional pain, this manual directed aid workers on how to read children's nonverbal signs of communication, including their bodily comportment and hand and facial gestures. CCI approached all children as fundamentally undeveloped subjects, and it identified language and communication as the major area where street children were undeveloped and required adult assistance. The manual claimed that because street life was so traumatic for them, street children could not express their own authentic desires or clearly articulate their experiences of pain. As a mode of aiding the street child, the manual suggested aid workers excavate children's feelings by asking certain questions or reading their bodies for signs of trauma. In sum, the manual promoted a set of expectations for aid workers that deepened their biomedical authority with street children and reified the supposed dependency children have on adults, especially with respect to language and the supposed "inner" pain that accompanies homelessness. The assumption, implicit throughout the manual, supposed a passive child and active clinician, seeing children's own actions as possible only through the aid worker's empowerment.

Both of CCI's medical manuals served as vehicles for the promotion of new global medical aid logics and practices in Egypt. They provided insights into how the organization defined street children's suffering and subsequently trained local workers to intervene accordingly. A glimpse into each manual suggests that, over all, the organization approached street children as physically and emotionally pathologized and dependent individuals. Conversely, the medical humanitarian encounter is imagined as one in which power and authority move singularly from adult aid worker to suffering street child. For instance, suggestions indicating practitioners should "give the child some power" pointed to practitioners' assumed position as the more powerful or active subject. In addition, the degree to which the practitioner should "help children raise questions," pointed towards the manner in which children were thought to depend on adults in order to communicate their own "inner" feelings. Together these standardized medical policies drove medical aid protocol in CCI's mobile clinic and were meant to guide the practices of its aid workers.

ENTANGLEMENTS OF AID: GENDER, CLASS, AND SHARED PRECARITY

Ramy, a twenty-two-year-old aid worker, who sat next to me one evening as we traveled through the city in the mobile clinic, was one of two low-level aid workers from CCI's shelter who joined Dr. Mohamad on his nightly patrols. "You know, the problem with Egypt is this—a very small population has everything," he complained. "The rest has nothing. We are a class society." CCI aid workers like Ramy did more than just help provide care for street children. They confronted the material and social realities of poverty zones in the city and became intimate with the plight of the urban poor. They were familiar with Cairo's worn-out pavements, dilapidated sidewalks, garbage-laden bridge underpasses, and overcrowded parking lots. Moreover, they regularly encountered the police in these sites and, in their encounters, had to negotiate their presence alongside local residents and street children. Sometimes this negotiation took the form of paying the police officers bribes; at other times, it meant avoiding the police entirely.

Most of CCI's shelter workers hailed from the working-class Giza neighborhood where the shelter was located. The majority were young men who also worked other part-time jobs in order to meet monthly expenses and save for future aspirations, such education or marriage. Two of the oldest boys from CCI's shelter usually rode along with us in order to assist in clinic work or enjoy a night out, away from the monotony and routines of the shelter. That night, young Islam and Rabʿ joined us and were chatting loudly in their seats the entire time. Much of the ride in the mobile clinic was spent in traffic as we traveled through city en route to one of several alternating mobile clinic stops. In order to pass the time during these extended drives, aid workers and street boys quipped about their shared male urban disenfranchisement and commented on politics. In these moments, aid workers situated themselves alongside street children in a permeable and fluid social relationship. Rather than an aid worker/aid recipient dichotomy, they understood their subjectivities as mingled together, sharing political claims against more powerful groups, and spoke about themselves as a kin network rooted at the shelter experiencing the same struggles.

The following vignette, taken from my field notes that night, offers a glimpse into these relational entanglements of aid. I was seated in a front seat near an open window when Ramy made his comment about Egypt being a "class society." He sat to my right and offered me a cigarette before lighting one up for himself. Samir, the clinic driver, was notoriously fast and erratic on the roads. It was ten o'clock in the evening. He wove rapidly through traffic as foggy air hit my face with accelerated force. It was summer and the heat was suffocating, even that late at night. The familiar scent of diesel fuel mixed with garbage alerted me that we were close to our destination—a clinic stop in the northern suburb of

Shubra al Khaima, an area that flourished during the industrial boom in Egypt's Nasserist era. Shubra al Khaima developed into a major center for commerce, and today, it remains a vibrant hub for commercial exchange and street vending. At its main metro stop, rows of wooden carts overflowing with clothes, housewares, sunglasses, and shoes for sale flanked the streets. It was an important clinic stop because bands of street children and youth worked the streets where shoppers strolled and socialized. Attracting patients at this stop was effortless due to the sheer number of children around, and Dr. Mohamad worked the location until the early morning hours.

As the mobile clinic crept closer to our final destination, Ramy continued with a string of critiques about corruption, injustice, and unethical politicians in Egypt. I listened attentively as he blamed the government for plundering Egypt's wealth, wealth that could have assisted the masses, average people like him. Abdou sat behind us. He was another aid worker from the shelter who was in his twenties. Abdou echoed Ramy's criticisms. As Ramy spoke, he nodded his head in agreement while playing classical Arabic music on his cell phone. The music kept Islam and Rabi` entertained and energetic throughout the ride.

Suddenly, while we were stopped in a traffic jam, a teenage street boy in a worn-out *galabiya* (male robe) approached the mobile clinic and yelled that he was selling mint leaves (*na'na*). Ramy and Abdou ignored him at first, but the eager young vendor persisted. He peered into the van, banged on our window, and vigorously shook a large bunch of mint leaves at our window. Abdou stood up from his seat, seemingly annoyed by the vendor's persistence, and pointed to the shiny black Mercedes rolling next to us on the streets, "You picked the wrong car! Go to Mr. Mercedes!" This outburst generated waves of laughter from Ramy, Islam, and Rabi', who found the joke appropriate and timely. The street vendor was trying to sell to former street boys and working-class aid workers instead of the obvious target—the driver of a Mercedes. The joke signaled the shared experience of the street vendor and the young men in the mobile clinic. In suggesting that the vendor sell to the other car, Abdou had marked his group as distinct from the apparently wealthy Mercedes driver. Abdou's joke situated clinic workers, former street boys, and the street vendor in the same—even if hierarchal—condition of urban disenfranchisement when juxtaposed against elite classes. It was just as much a statement on inequality as it was an impeccably timed joke at the expense of the young street vendor. In contrast to how aid workers are approached in CCI policy—as powerful subjects tasked with helping vulnerable children—the incident described above wove Abdou, Ramy, Islam, Rabi', and the young street vendor together in a mutual situation of masculine precarity, and within the same social and political context.

In writing about the work of the United Nations Relief and Works Agency for Palestine Refugees (UNRWA) and the United Nations High Commission for Refugees (UNHCR), Ilana Feldman has also traced the ways in which humanitarian subject positions are much less distinct than we would presume. As she notes, "the boundaries between the categories of provider and recipient are fuzzy," in the bulk of humanitarian work that takes place today.[15] This is because humanitarian staff are mostly themselves members of recipient communities. At CCI, intermittent volunteer work and medical training sessions were run by foreign-born professionals, but the majority of the organization's aid work on the streets, and the work I observed most closely while in the field, was conducted by local Egyptian employees. This was especially the case with the mobile clinic. Mobile clinic workers were entirely local due to the rigorous nature of the fieldwork and the late-night outings that were required of all clinic staff. Clinic workers were not afforded the same "cultural distance" and "affective neutrality" foreign aid workers ostensibly experience.[16] Rather, they confront recipient needs up close and personally and negotiate the same social and economic conditions in their own everyday lives.

DR. MOHAMAD

Low-level clinic workers were not the only mobile clinic aid providers who had to manage their own economic conditions and who saw their lives as interwoven with those of child aid recipients. Humanitarian doctors had obligations and responsibilities that shaped their work commitments and relationships as well. In my interviews with Dr. Mohamad, he often conveyed deep concern over his future due to his economic and professional aspirations. During our first nightly patrol, I asked him how he became interested in working for CCI's mobile clinic. In speaking about his life up to that point, Dr. Mohamad echoed many young, educated professionals I spoke with in Cairo who aspired to a better livelihood and more prosperous future. He was a government physician and general practitioner by day—a job that earned him a very modest income—and worked in CCI's mobile clinic at night. He sought this second, evening job in the international humanitarian sector with CCI in order to save enough money to secure his prospects for a future marriage, the economic burdens of which would fall on his family. He lived with his parents and a sister in a spacious apartment located in one of Cairo's sought-after middle-class neighborhoods. By working days and evenings, he hoped to purchase an apartment nearby for his own future family. Living with his family allowed him to contribute to his household's comfort while saving a considerable amount of money. Dr. Mohamad also hoped to return to school at some point in the future and further his education by delving into a more specialized medical field. The extra income generated from evening work with CCI helped him secure funds for these future goals. He confessed to me that the income he earned from working for CCI was far more substantial than that from any local medical aid jobs available to him.

Despite the economic benefits that accompanied medical aid work at CCI, Dr. Mohamad still articulated his interventions with street children through ethical terms. He spoke about the work as a humanitarian commitment, an obligation he carried out for both street children and the country as a whole. "I have to do something about the problem," was a statement I heard frequently when Dr. Mohamad spoke about street children as one of Egypt's greatest social problems. For him and many other workers at CCI, the sight of children living and working on the streets was a moral stain on Egyptian national consciousness. It was a sign of society's collective economic and social failure, and signified a crisis that needed remedy, in any form possible, since street children embodied the upsetting of familial norms and codes.[17] In this respect, Dr. Mohamad understood his work as having immediate, if limited, effects for individual children as well as the imagined future nation.

Unlike other mobile clinic workers like Abdou and Ramy, Dr. Mohamad was instantly differentiated as a middle-class professional in the areas where clinic work took place. He always dressed in fashionable collared shirts and sported stylish dark-framed glasses. His well-groomed hair was slicked back and neat, held in place by copious amounts of hair gel. His frequent use of English words when describing medical procedures to aid workers or children solidified his middle-class, expert status and garnered him respect and authority. Yet, like child recipients and low-level aid workers, he was also embedded in a set of struggles and obligations. Like them, he was constrained by future aspirations, and these aspirations shaped his present-day decision-making practices. Although less violent and physically conspicuous, they also left material marks upon his body and produced health-related consequences in his life. Working a double medical shift every day and night in the public and international aid healthcare sectors left him perpetually sleep-deprived. Exhaustion was a daily fact for Dr. Mohamad. On some nights, before our mobile aid shift began, he locked himself in the back of the clinic for a necessary nap. We waited patiently outside the clinic during these times, waiting for him to awaken as we played games with children or passed out coloring books and snacks. The children understood that aid work was taxing for Dr. Mohamad. He sometimes treated dozens of children for hours on end without a single break. One night, as he napped, I mingled with children near the clinic and discovered their deep sense of sympathy for Dr. Mohamad and their awareness of his physical limitations. A young boy was kicking an empty soda can while waiting for the clinic to open. Searching for a subject to start a conversation, I asked if he knew where the doctor was. With a gleaming smile, he pointing to the back of the clinic and warned me to keep quiet so that Dr. Mohamad could sleep. "The doctor needs to sleep," he said. "He's very tired. You have to wait for him." His comment conveyed a sense of respect for Dr. Mohamad's time, but also a level of care and concern for his bodily welfare. It took me by surprise. Abdou was standing nearby and overheard the exchange. I asked if he had noticed how concerned the young boy was about Dr. Mohamad's nap. Abdou immediately explained the mutual care linking Dr. Mohamad and the children. With a tinge of admiration, he observed that Dr. Mohamad was a committed humanitarian who was driven by his "heart." He gestured to the young boy, saying, "You can tell he loves them. In order to do this kind of work, it has to come from the heart."

In an ethnography of infectious disease in Zambia, Jean Hunleth has shown how children empathize with, care for, and even manage pharmaceutical regimens for their adult family members who are suffering from tuberculosis or HIV.[18] This means that children, and not only adults, understand and shape biomedical practice in their own particular ways and with the hope of achieving what, for them, would be beneficial social outcomes. The compassion children expressed for Dr. Mohamad reflected a similar instance of children caring for adults. Yet the compassion for Dr. Mohamad expressed by children at CCI went beyond the household relationships Hunleth has studied. It showed that children could care for adults in clinical settings, outside of their homes and with nonrelatives. Indeed, children's care and compassion for adults represents a more expansive and diverse social field than many of our studies of global aid have accounted for thus far.

MOBILE MEDICAL ENCOUNTERS

Dr. Mohamad wiped sweat from his brow for the third time while preparing some bandages as we organized supplies. It was summer, the mobile clinic lacked air conditioning, and the heat was oppressive. We were in Shubra al Khaima again, discussing the clinic's broad outcomes, when he brought up the topic of medical statistics. "The most common problem for children we see in this clinic is gastroenteritis from stomach infections. You know, from very bad food conditions." A data log hung conspicuously on a clipboard at the entrance of the clinic's examination room. When Dr. Mohamad conducted a physical examination, or checked vital signs on a child patient, an aid worker documented the child's name, age, ailment, and the course of medical action taken on the data log. Shuffling through the papers that were on the clipboard, he held it up for me to see and continued, "Look at this. It shows the list from last month." Leaning over from my seat, I skimmed through the pile of disheveled papers. The top sheet featured a list handwritten in Arabic identifying "stomach infections" as the most common form of child illness treated in the clinic. Under it was a line that read "infected wounds." These wounds, he claimed, were commonly caused by car accidents or street fights. Dr. Mohamad elaborated these realities of street life, describing how street children got nails or shards of glass lodged in their feet all of the time because their flip-flops—the most inexpensive shoe they could own—lacked protective soles. "The kids then run in and out of traffic. They sell things and wipe windows with these shoes. It's very dangerous for them," he lamented.

In fact, in the clinic all summer, Dr. Mohamad treated countless foot wounds, first by applying a heavy dose of Betadine (a cheap antiseptic) to the wound and then by securing a clean bandage around it. These encounters took only a few minutes to complete, but they were numerous and occupied the bulk of our nightly work. My usual job was to cut bandages or surgical tape in preparation for these procedures. Witnessing countless children enter the clinic with the same healthcare predicament—a nail or piece of glass lodged in their foot—revealed the dangerous patterns shaping their lives and vividly illustrated the hazardous urban streets that threatened tiny exposed feet. Throat and chest infections were the third most common ailment Dr. Mohamad treated in the clinic. These problems resulted from a mixture of urban pollution and children's incessant cigarette smoking. These throat and chest ailments were particularly pronounced among boys and young men who visited the clinic. As mentioned earlier, smoking for street boys is a sign of masculinity, it garners respect on the streets and signifies manhood. It also staves off hunger. Boys smoked heavily on the streets, sometimes beginning as early as age five or six.

Inadequate footwear, street labor, pollution, and masculine norms that propel so-called dangerous habits—these were the primary causes of wounds and illnesses experienced by aid recipients, the conditions that prompted them to visit the clinic and receive medical care. Just as Kleinman noted how the experience of illness reflects our unique biographies, as well as the social situations and webs of relationships we are embedded in, Dr. Mohamad considered street children's suffering, their "illness narratives," as inseparable from their life histories and economic struggles.[19] Dr. Mohamad referenced CCI's medical-social approach as a helpful guide in delivering treatment to street children. For him, the approach recognized the relationship between children and their environment, and the ways in which street life shaped individual child health. But he reminded me that despite his delivering optimum humanitarian care, the kind CCI promoted, and after giving children sound medical advice about how to stay safe and remain clean on the streets, children often disregarded his words. He was an adult and an authority figure after all, and notwithstanding the care and respect they shared for each other, street children did not "trust" any adult authority figures, including him. "Then who do they trust," I interjected after hearing this, wondering how children as young as five managed daily life on the streets without adult assistance. "They listen mostly only to their friends," he said.

To mitigate this distrust, Dr. Mohamad constantly negotiated his authority with street children, guiding medical encounters while conceding to children's desires and requests. Drawing on local knowledge of the city and his own experiences with the police, he improvised his medical practices in order to achieve the most successful outcomes for clinic patients. Success, for him, entailed a range of results, from adhering to formal CCI policy to making some kind of expert intervention in children's physical welfare, whether it be temporary and limited, or social rather than medical. The following three ethnographic vignettes from the mobile clinic illustrate this kind of delicate negotiation by Dr. Mohamad. Each interaction captures a different unintended consequence of mobile aid with street boys. Together, they demonstrate how formal global medical aid scripts and goals get reconstituted and transformed, locally, as a result of aid recipient agency and Cairo's political and historical context. As the encounters played out, I tried to maintain my commitment to Dr. Mohamad and CCI, which was to assist in the management of children in the clinic and follow formalized rights-based care. Yet just as in chapter one, this position situated me as an adult authority figure with children, and therefore marked me as a non-neutral subject, even if I spent most of the time simply seated near the examination table handing Dr. Mohamad supplies or observing in silence.

PAIN AND MEDICAL NONCOMPLIANCE

Amir was eleven years old and a regular patient at the Shubra al Khaima stop. When I first met him, Dr. Mohamad had already been treating him in CCI's mobile clinic for a year, for symptoms ranging from minor infections to general checkups. Clinic workers knew Amir's history quite well. He had been working on the streets around the metro stop since the age of nine, when he left his household. This was also the age when he began smoking cigarettes. After entering the clinic, he greeted Abdou and me with a firm handshake and broad smile, but embraced Dr. Mohamad for several long seconds, a greeting that reflected their shared affection and familiarity with each other. Amir settled onto the examination table without hesitation, his thin legs dangled off the edge. Dr. Mohamad checked his vital signs and asked a set of routine questions about his health and overall status, saying, "Are you having any problems right now?" Amir quickly responded that he suffered from a recurring dry cough and sore throat. These were causing him tremendous pain, which, once the examination was under way and his vital signs checked, he expressed to us by grabbing his throat and speaking loudly in a hoarse, broken voice.

Looking into his throat, Dr. Mohamad questioned Amir about his ongoing smoking habits, which everyone in the clinic was aware of. Amir deflected the question away from his smoking by asking Dr. Mohamad for a bottle of cough syrup so that he could simply be on his way. Dr. Mohamad explained to Amir that he had an infection, one that required antibiotic pills, and that the cough syrup would not be enough to cure his condition or alleviate the pain. To this, Amir shook his head in defiance and expressed aversion to the antibiotics. He responded by repeating that he wanted the syrup, because it was the only medication that would produce immediate results. Craning his neck, he looked up directly into Dr. Mohamad eyes and said that "pills take too long," and what he wanted was immediate relief.

Dr. Mohamad sighed and pulled a white box of antibiotics out of the medicine cabinet, along with a small bottle of herbal cough syrup. He placed both in Amir's small hands, but not before proceeding to educate Amir on how antibiotics work: first by traveling through the blood, then by traveling to the throat, and finally curing the infection and providing lasting relief as oppose to the syrup's temporary effects. Amir listened to this medical lesson with a smile, but halfway into it he shook his head in defiance and again asked for the syrup. His willful giggling and head shaking during Dr. Mohamad's explanation was a sign of his resistance and medical noncompliance. Dr. Mohamad continued to attempt to educate Amir, his frustration with Amir growing more visible by the second. Eventually, he ended the encounter by sending Amir on his way with both medications.

Having witnessed the subtle sparring between Amir and Dr. Mohamad, I asked if Amir would eventually take the pills, throw them away, or if he would consume the entire bottle of cough syrup all at once in order to experience its intoxicating effects. Dr. Mohamad believed any of these things might occur. "Carrying a bottle around the city is troublesome for street children. They need to travel light, so he might drink the syrup all at once." We were both unsure about how Amir would consume the medications he had received, or whether his painful throat infection would be cured. Dr. Mohamad said he strongly doubted that Amir would heed his advice about taking the pills. My unease at this unknown outcome and my concern for Amir's welfare undoubtedly showed on my face. Dr. Mohamad attempted to reassure me by smiling, shrugging his shoulders, and claiming that this was business as usual with street children. In educating Amir and providing him with medication, he had reached the limits of his humanitarian intervention with Amir. He softly mumbled, "What else can I do?"

Gendered Solidarity and Police Violence

Like Amir, Walid was a regular patient of the mobile clinic at the Shubra al Khaima stop and knew all the mobile clinic aid workers very well. Workers told me he was nineteen years old when I met him. This meant that he did not fall into the formal category of "street child" as laid down in CCI policy—a person under the age of eighteen. Still, having procured care from Dr. Mohamad on and off for over two years, he regularly used the clinic, viewing it as a valuable source of assistance and male sociality. Workers welcomed him accordingly, happy to extend their work with older street children like him beyond the normative age of "childhood." Typical of homeless boys who have lived on the streets for long periods of time, Walid was missing several front teeth. This showed in the big smile he put on immediately after he entered the clinic one night. Although the summer heat was intense, he wore a faded brown leather jacket over a ripped T-shirt and jeans. Thick, wavy brown hair hung over his face, and at over six feet tall, he had to duck to make his way into the clinic and onto the examination table. Extensive greetings were exchanged between him and Dr. Mohamad. Moments later, Abdou and Ramy joined in on the meeting and relished hearing about Walid's life since the last time he had visited the clinic.

Aid workers have grown fondly attached to Walid over the years. They believed he was a brave young man, and were especially proud of his success at avoiding police detention. Despite the recent rights-based amendments to Egypt's new child law, the police in Cairo continued to detain, intimidate, and physically abuse young men living on the streets. To avoid this, Walid had repeatedly inflicted wounds across his own chest and arms with a knife or razor when confronted by a threatening police officer. Although painful, this worked for Walid and, according to Ramy and Abdou, kept him from being detained. On the examination table, Walid lifted his T-shirt to reveal a tapestry of self-inflicted wounds, showing off what to him were signs of his manhood. I had never seen anything like Walid's scars before—razor blade marks scattered across his arms and torso. As Dr. Mohamad examined the scars, he explained how they served an important function on the streets. To my surprise, he did not dole advice out to Walid about the dangers of creating such wounds. Instead, he identified danger as lying with the police. He justified the scars by explaining how the police sought to avoid accountability for "human rights abuses." If a young man appeared to be bleeding, they passed him by so as to avoid responsibility for his suffering or death. For Dr. Mohamad, the state (*al hakuma*) produced the scars; its concern lay not in decreasing deaths on the streets but in decreasing collective public outrage and uprisings against it. Walid had been arrested and subjected to police abuse before. He had learned, in his eight years of living on the streets, that he could successfully mobilize his own body in this way in confrontations with the police to avoid detention.

By cutting himself, Walid used his body as a vehicle of "rhetorical performance" with the police, creating a spectacle of wounds in order to secure his own safety and freedom.[20] The scars ran in multiple directions across his chest and arms, some fresh, some ancient, but each narrated a history of gender and class violence. In the clinic, Dr. Mohamad and Walid spoke about these wounds as a sign of masculine bravery and as a means of resistance to an illegitimate state. For them, they were a testament to the scale of terror young homeless men face on the streets. The night he visited the clinic, Walid did not have an urgent medical condition that needed attention. Rather, he had come simply to update aid workers on events in his life. As Walid socialized with us, Ramy and Abdou gave him information about where to travel in the city. They detailed the areas where they thought the police were less present, pointing Walid towards these safer neighborhoods. It had been twenty minutes since his arrival when Dr. Mohamad began a routine check of Walid's vital signs. After exchanging more friendly banter, and before sending him off for the night, he handed Walid a gift bag, along with a small stack of ointments, bandages, and mild painkillers. Walid left just as Dr. Mohamad affectionately said, "And remember don't smoke!" It was the one piece of advice he knew Walid would likely ignore.

Walid received vital biomedical care for his physical wounds in the clinic. But to him and aid workers, these wounds were necessary, in that they helped him secure better health by avoiding police detention and, in turn, extensive physical, emotional, and sexual abuse. Mobile clinic workers regarded Walid's self-inflicted wounds and long-term struggle with the police as legitimate. Along with medical aid for these wounds, they gave him other forms of assistance that helped him resist the police—including advice about where to be in the city to remain safe. Through their repeated clinic encounters, Walid and aid workers developed lasting bonds of male affection and solidarity.

After he left the clinic, stories about Walid's endurance and bravery continued to circulate in the clinic. Ramy and Abdou emphasized these stories in my presence, perhaps because I was the only woman present during nightly patrols. In this gendered politics of the body, Walid seemed fearless and above immediate pain. The cuts and wounds he produced served a greater purpose, one that lay beyond the present. The threat of police detention prevailed over the pain of these razor cuts. We see in his story how street children's pain and suffering is embedded in social relations that extend beyond individual embodiment. Indeed, Walid's wounds were "social wounds" that spoke most clearly to his status as a social agent and object of state power.[21] His class and gender entanglements with oppressive urban structures—particularly the police—prompted a form of violence as an act of resistance. Wounds, here, were more than a source of pain and trauma, as stated in CCI policy. They were productive, an avenue towards safety and dignity, even if painful.

Confronting Poverty in the City

In a context of urban poverty, where public healthcare structures were minimal or nonexistent, it was difficult to ensure that street children were the only recipients who drew upon CCI's mobile medical clinic for healthcare. With its stark white façade and imposing read letters, the clinic was difficult to ignore. By patrolling streets where children congregated and worked, the clinic was present in areas of the city where disenfranchisement and need were widespread. Other vulnerable populations, and not only street children, recognized the mobile clinic as a valuable provider of quick and free healthcare. In this respect, the mobile clinic did more in Cairo than what CCI policy intended it to do. While in some respects it remained limited in the care that it provided for street children, it surpassed its stated aims by providing vital healthcare to other groups.

One night, we parked the clinic at a vibrant intersection in Muhandasin, a newly gentrified area of the city. Fashionable cafés, clothing shops, and restaurants lined the streets where children labored and lived, seeking out middle-class consumers for fast cash. At approximately one o'clock in the morning, during one of our slower hours, a young woman who was holding a baby and accompanied by two older women, presumably relatives, approached the mobile clinic. We soon learned that she was desperately seeking assistance for her newborn. She passed the infant through the clinic's back window and pleaded to Dr. Mohamad for treatment. All three women wore long black *abayas* (robes) with matching black headscarves. According to Dr. Mohamad, this indicated their status as urban poor. After quickly examining the baby, Dr. Mohamad passed her back through the window and back into the arms of the mother. As she rocked the baby to one side, Dr. Mohamad passed her several packets of medication and directed her on how to give the treatment to the baby. The three women then exchanged a string of religious messages of gratitude. With impassioned voices, they thanked Dr. Mohamad for his assistance and prayed that God "would be with him."[22]

Once they were out of sight, Dr. Mohamad observed that the baby had chickenpox, a condition he had treated in the clinic before. However, the fleeting medical encounter he had just had with the women and the baby remained off the books. As such, it was dependent on his humanitarian sense of compassion, his discretionary judgment, and his willingness to treat vulnerable groups that were not the clinic's target population. Here, mobile medical aid extended beyond formal policy, reaching a broader urban poor population, including a woman who was not formally "homeless" but who nevertheless needed healthcare assistance for her suffering infant. Dr. Mohamad considered the encounter his humanitarian obligation. He justified such exchanges by suggesting that other groups required assistance just as much as street children, perhaps even more. His voice signaled distress as he shook his head and remarked, "These women have nowhere else to go to get medicine for their babies."

DOING MORE BUT NOT ENOUGH

The three cases presented in this chapter, gleaned from my time in CCI's mobile medical clinic, form a triad of illness narratives that were distinct yet folded into one another in Cairo's bustling urban landscape. Each case reflects how care in the mobile medical clinic is at once emancipatory and limited for both aid workers and recipients. Each story illustrates how poverty and homelessness left lasting marks upon mobile child bodies, and how the clinic offered a temporary resolution to those marks. The vignettes mostly demonstrate how within the mobile clinic, formal aid policy was either challenged or reconstituted and remade because it fell short of recipient expectations or exceeded them.[23] In the mobile clinic, many children practiced some degree of medical noncompliance. Moreover, they openly expressed their own feelings of pain. Power moved both ways in the medical aid encounter, as well as compassion, care, and solidarity. These on-the-ground practices dramatically unsettled CCI's formal global aid policy and shattered key assumptions in policy about street children's inherent passivity and inability to communicate. The patients discussed in this chapter, contrary to what the policy asserted, did not require a medical practitioner's help in "unearthing" inner experiences or feelings of pain. At the same time, Dr. Mohamad's authority had its limits in the clinic; he was left to improvise care and alter his practices to accommodate patient desires. Medical authority, during these mobile medical aid encounters, was complex and malleable.

Some aid recipients, like Walid, experienced police violence and the threat of detention regularly on the streets. They have come to use the clinic for much more than biomedical aid. For them, the mobile clinic was a safe haven and a source of temporary relief from police oppression. Other vulnerable groups learned to recognize CCI's mobile clinic as a valuable resource in the city, a space where they could receive free, efficient healthcare in the absence of other forms of assistance. In order to procure care, these groups hedged their bets on Dr. Mohamad's sense of compassion towards them. Their reliance on global aid actors like humanitarian doctors reminds us how widespread and all-encompassing bodily vulnerability is in cities around the world where free and public healthcare has been dismantled or significantly reduced. All of these aid-driven social entanglements, as they occurred in and through CCI's mobile medical clinic, presented aid workers with ethical and material challenges for which they had to make decisions on their own, and outside of formal policy guidelines.

If mobile medical aid is the embodiment of the humanitarian gesture, as Peter Redfield has claimed in his work on mobile aid, then mobile care enacted in the name of suffering children represents the quintessential expression of care from global aid organizations.[24] Mobile medicine has long been considered the quickest and most precise response to widespread healthcare crises, refracting back onto its history as an outgrowth of war and an urgent necessity to save human lives. But the experiences I witnessed in CCI's mobile clinic demonstrate just how this form of care is enacted in contexts that produce grounded tensions. These tensions exist beyond formal policy and must be continually negotiated by aid workers and aid recipients. They suggest we not only look at individual child bodies as the site of intervention, but beyond them, into the social conditions that produced the suffering and children's attempts to mitigate them, including labor practices, police violence, public discrimination against the homeless, and disintegrating social services resulting from neoliberal reforms.[25] If we do, the boundaries between children's bodily wounds and social wounds become more porous, even inseparable, and the paradoxes—the benefits and limitations—of mobile medical aid as a response to suffering come into full view.[26]

Chapter 3

(IN)VISIBLE WOUNDS

CCI APPROACHED ALL STREET CHILDREN AS EMOTIONAL SUFFERERS who were traumatized. As such they were in need of mental healthcare in addition to physical care.[1] Like other prominent global aid organizations that were active across the region at the time of my fieldwork, psychiatric interventions (sometimes labeled psycho-social programs) for street children were rapidly expanding within CCI. Along with physical suffering, street children were described in global aid policy that promoted this work as subjects who carried the burden of invisible wounds, or psychic trauma—the hidden yet enduring result of life lived on harsh and unforgiving streets without a family. CCI was a leader in recognizing the emotional health of street children across the Middle East since the 1990s. The street children's shelter in Giza hosted programs around child mental health, and conducted psychiatric examinations on children that foregrounded their emotions as a key area for medical intervention. With language inciting compassion for children's inner pain and pathologies, CCI considered its free psychiatric and psycho-social programs a valuable service for individual children and a means to help craft a safer and healthier nation in the future.

This chapter explores what global psychiatric aid does for street children and aid workers at CCI's shelter. Although all street children were constructed in CCI policy as emotional sufferers carrying invisible wounds in the same, universalized ways, and through biomedical frameworks of health, I quickly learned, in tracing this care in practice, that not all children received ongoing care from the organization's psychiatrist. Rather, aid workers identified "problem" boys as the ideal subjects for psychiatric intervention. The fear, as aid workers put it to me when I inquired about this, was that boys would likely "explode" if their trauma was left untreated and buried inside them. This would then create violence and chaos within the shelter community and, eventually, outside of it. Although psychiatry was framed in the language of compassion and rights in CCI policy, on the ground child psychiatric care engendered an unequal distribution of aid, one that marked some boys as potential threats to the shelter community. In some cases, this status resulted in their exclusion from CCI's humanitarian shelter. The paradoxical status ascribed to problem boys, of emotional victim yet potential threat, further deepened street boys' disenfranchisement by more closely associating them to discourses of violence, danger, and unruly masculinity.[2]

On a crisp and cool January morning, I accompanied Mahmud and Hassan, two boys living at CCI, to their monthly psychiatric appointment. We departed the shelter at 9:00 a.m. and arrived downtown at the organization's psychiatric clinic over an hour later. Mahmud, fourteen, and Hassan, eight, barely spoke on our long ride to the clinic. After our arrival, they sat quietly on plastic chairs in the waiting room and barely acknowledged me, with exhaustion apparent on each of their faces. Sensing the boys were uninterested in conversation, I sat on the opposite side of the waiting room, where twenty-four-year old Ahmed, the CCI aid worker who drove us to the clinic, fiddled with the channels on a clunky television set. The clinic appeared eerily sterile. It had high ceilings, bare walls, and lacked heating, making the room incredibly chilly. I rubbed my hands together for warmth and focused on the show Ahmed chose to watch, a popular Syrian soap opera that blared colorful imagery and dramatic dialogue across the room. Mahmud and Hassan shivered from the cold as well and simply stared at the television screen. The mood in the room was solemn as we sat, silently, for what felt like countless minutes while waiting for Dr. Mona, CCI's paid child psychiatrist. Mahmud and Hassan were brought to this clinic once a month for follow-up therapy appointments. During these visits, they engaged in talk therapy with Dr. Mona and she monitored their progress with medication. Dr. Mona strove to teach the boys how to talk about their problems and think of themselves as children who had suffered psychic trauma, but who could, with active participation in psychotherapy, become psychologically rehabilitated, stable, and healthy.

The anthropologists Didier Fassin and Richard Rechtman have labeled the form of biomedical intervention Dr. Mona practiced at CCI "humanitarian psychiatry." They consider this work a contemporary practice that emerged in the 1980s, when organizations first incorporated psychic care into global humanitarian programs. Since then, humanitarian psychiatry has garnered wide-scale attention as a legitimate, ethical response to human suffering born of war, crisis, or extreme poverty. The logics undergirding humanitarian psychiatry, as Fassin and Rechtman have noted, assert that tragedies—from natural disasters to political violence—leave lasting marks on both human bodies and minds. But where bodily wounds in crisis zones call attention to the need for medical doctors, psychic trauma necessitates the deployment of psychiatrists, therapists, and mental health experts.[3] However in Egypt, local conceptualizations of biomedical health stigmatize mental illness and the use of psychiatric or psychological assistance. Seeking emotional care from a biomedical healthcare professional in a clinical setting, rather than a family member or religious figure, is rare, even among the middle and elite classes. How then is global psychiatric care practiced and received at CCI? I was especially curious to learn more about how psychiatric aid was understood in practice by children and Dr. Mona as I sat with Mahmud and Hassan in the clinic's waiting room.

Usually rambunctious at the shelter, now Hassan remained still in his chair. Mahmud appeared sleepier and more dejected by the minute. With eyes still fixed on the television screen, Mahmud finally mumbled, "I hate coming here." He kicked his flip-flops, which had fallen off, with his right foot. I turned to Ahmed, our driver, for an explanation as to why both boys appeared so distraught since we arrived at the clinic. He just shrugged and indicated that this was "normal." He talked about the numerous trips he made to this clinic with children, and explained that they never enjoyed psychiatric visits because they were always forced to think about "bad memories," especially their past family problems. He expected Mahmud and Hassan to resist their appointments with Dr. Mona. Their behavior was merely part of the rehabilitation process, a process that was "good" for children even if they struggled with it. Roughly twenty more minutes elapsed before Mahmud was finally called in first for his appointment. Hassan and I watched as he disappeared behind closed doors for his seemingly dreaded, yet necessary, according to Ahmed, therapy session.

In the past, both boys had been diagnosed by Dr. Mona as suffering from the clinical conditions of "depression" and "mood disorders." As such they were obligated to participate in CCI's psychiatric program as long as they remained at the shelter. In other words, psychiatric care was compulsory, not voluntary, for the children Dr. Mona diagnosed as suffering from clinical disorders.[4] Dr. Mona and other CCI aid workers believed that social and economic factors produced the trauma that led to these disorders, but that psychiatric intervention would uncover the hidden trauma and initiate the healing of emotional wounds.

At the shelter, trauma was linked to problematic behavior, and aid workers considered Mahmud and Hassan among their most "problematic" children. The boys were notorious for challenging adult authority as well as shelter norms about childhood. In addition, both boys were considered unstable in ways that threatened the health and safety of others in the community. Mahmud was the oldest boy housed at the shelter and one of its first recipients, having joined the shelter when it opened its doors in 2004. Workers had difficulty keeping him at the shelter. He repeatedly left in order to work and rejoin a group of friends he had previously acquired on the streets. Workers strove to assist Mahmud in crafting a healthy, productive life, but they never knew when he would return. His sojourns could last anywhere from a few weeks to several months. Mahmud was tall for his age and always had a quiet disposition. While aid workers lauded his reserve and respectful attitude, they complained about his independence and tendency to disappear.

By contrast, young Hassan was notorious for his loud, angry fits and for initiating fights with other children. For this reason, aid workers labeled him a "trouble maker" (*kulu mashakil*). Workers viewed his mischievous behavior as owing to his childhood abandonment. His impoverished mother could no longer care for him at age five and simply left him at the front gate of the shelter. Workers understood this narrative as legitimating his uncontrollable outbursts but also his need for psychiatric intervention, and for biological normalization. In workshops held at the shelter, they learned that talk therapy and medication could bring him closer to the end goal of rehabilitation, to eventual "psychological health" (*al-siha al-nafsiya*).

I was in Dr. Mona's office that morning with two boys who were considered the shelter's most "problematic" children. Yet, as I came to learn, their gender wasn't a coincidence. In policy, psychiatry was framed as a legitimate intervention for all street children. This meant that all children at the shelter were, in theory, emotionally vulnerable and traumatized due to their homelessness. However, at CCI, boys were disproportionately approached as ideal psychiatric subjects in ways girls were not. I strove to understand the underpinnings of this unequal distribution of care on the ground, and discovered that local perceptions about gender and violence on the streets were central to it. In linking former street boys' inner wounds to the specter of social violence, aid workers hoped to biologically "stabilize" them, which would then ensure social stability. They spoke about problem boys in ways suggesting that they embodied crisis, using words such as "explosion," "dangerous," and "unstable" to describe their behavior. Dr. Mona's nurse elaborated this point, commenting to me during an interview that, "Emotional disorders experienced by *these* [her emphasis] boys could easily explode into social instability."

As CCI aid workers considered some boys traumatized and potentially dangerous, all street girls were considered traumatized yet less threatening, or not threatening at all. As such they participated in other compulsory forms of emotional care at the shelter, including creative art therapy classes meant to unearth hidden feelings of trauma, or fitness and exercise sessions intended to positively alter their moods through physiological activity. While these differences in care practices overlapped for some children, in general boys remained the primary objects of psychiatric and psycho-pharmaceutical intervention. Dubbed trouble, problem, or difficult, these boys appeared to aid workers as dually vulnerable and threatening. The following pages explore this gendered condition, and its social effects, in greater length.

HOW GENDER SHAPES EMOTIONAL SUFFERING

An entire section of CCI's mission statement delved into the problem of street children's emotional suffering. It described how the organization dedicated substantial funds to child psychiatry and even launched a twenty-four-hour hotline for street children to dial in on if they needed emergency counseling. In colorful pamphlets, the organization promoted its psychiatric program with images of boys huddled together smiling widely. They appeared cooperative and joyful. In one image, a boy boasts a playful thumbs-up to the camera as his peers surround him in a warm embrace. Images such as these in humanitarian media, of vibrant, happy children, could be remarkably productive for organizations such as CCI. They help increase donor funds for aid programs by inciting sympathy for vulnerable children who also appear playful and innocent. As Mckenzie Wark has noted, humanitarian images like these circulate transnationally in a robust moral economy of international aid for the child. They affectively convey powerful "truths" about childhood innocence, distant suffering, and the purported successes of global humanitarian interventions.[5] But these "truths" stood in stark contrast to how Mahmud and Hassan experienced their psychiatric aid.

At CCI, emotional intervention—which included psychiatry but also a range of practices centered on children's trauma—was mandatory. Children were compelled to take part in emotional care if they wanted to live at the shelter and remain part of the community.

Despite the disproportionate usage of boys in the humanitarian media images I encountered, trauma care and psychiatric interventions were framed as ungendered aid practices in global aid policy. Policy discourses did not feature clear distinctions between street children's experiences of emotional pain or trauma, whether it be according to children's gender, age, or any other distinguishing factor. Yet the local responses to children's emotional health at CCI's shelter and in Dr. Mona's clinic were anything but universal and homogenous. Rather, care practices were contingent on gender, as well as a range of other social factors, including age, behavior, appearance, and a child's general demeanor. To aid workers at CCI, girls and boys demonstrated their trauma differently, and these differences mobilized different responses from them.[6]

Adult anxieties about poor boys from the streets and the threat they embody has been the subject of studies on cities across the global south.[7] In the United States, we have witnessed how healthcare policies and formal diagnoses of mentally ill persons reflected deep-seated social inequalities. The racialization of schizophrenia, for instance, as Jonathan Metzl has detailed, is a prominent case in point. Since the 1960s, so-called angry black masculinity in the United States has been seen as requiring psychiatric treatment because symptoms were believed to simultaneously threaten society as well as the subject's own sanity.[8] What this example of racial inequity has in common with my observations at CCI is the interpretation of biological conditions in terms of sociopolitical relations, and an attempt to manage future (imagined) stability through interventions that target vulnerable young male populations. At CCI, attempts to manage young, unruly masculine subjects showed up in aid documents workers produced about street children, such as personal histories and medical reports. Ironically, in order to construct these narrative truths about children's inner states, and in order to engage children in proper psychiatric care, aid workers had to see the signs of trauma on children's bodies. In other words, aid workers had to identify visible signs of emotional suffering. They had to recognize and care for these invisible wounds, but this required a significant amount of guesswork and interpretation. To accomplish this, aid workers drew equally on local understandings about the streets, gender, and age, and on their knowledge of standardized global aid policy and biomedical procedures. While their ultimate aim was to address trauma, and thereby alleviate children's emotional suffering, aid workers were positioned to make critical distinctions between children. This work ended up reproducing social inequalities for some children, especially boys like Mahmud and Hassan.[9]

TRAUMA, BODIES, AND A GENDERED SPECTRUM OF CARE

In my discussions with CCI aid workers and volunteers at the Giza children's shelter, I learned about what it meant to be a child *min al shariʿ* (from the streets). Many workers used this term casually when talking about individual children's life histories and the unfortunate circumstances that produced their homelessness and brought them to the shelter. For instance, when explaining why a particular child caused problems at the shelter or engaged in troublesome behavior, workers stated that children did such things because they were "from the streets." I heard countless explanations along the lines of "That child is quiet [or jealous, or craving attention] because they are *min al shariʿ*." In time, I learned that the meanings of *min al shariʿ* differed for aid workers according to a child's gender and age group, and these differences informed the compassion or discipline with which they treated children.

Important decisions were made at the shelter based on conceptualizations of what street life was like for each child, and these decisions—typically implemented quickly on the spot—had real consequences for children at the shelter. Was the child an active perpetrator of violence on the streets? Or was the child a victim of violence on the streets? How did the child's history affect other children at the shelter? These were some of the questions workers pondered when dealing with children's daily lives. Aid workers described all of the children as victims of forces beyond their control, including poverty, divorce, and police violence. But the older, teenage boys were also understood as suspects who could actively perpetrate violence (physical and sexual) against other children. They were viewed as more likely to cause lasting problems for workers and other children. The youngest girls, on the other hand, were framed in the conversations of aid workers as purely innocent or the passive potential victims of older male suspects. Compassion, exclusion, and punishment at the shelter were structured by aid workers around such shared ideas about gender, power, age, and violence.

One of the most important decisions tied to these gendered understandings of victimhood and violence had to do with entry into the shelter community. Because of the threat of violence and disruption they embodied, CCI did not admit all boys who sought to enter the shelter. Some were granted entry, while others were excluded, and there was a critical screening process that distinguished between the two. In general, workers' sense of compassion and local ideas about masculine violence drove decisions about entry. Here, as in other accounts of humanitarianism, gender and power intersected to exclude certain groups from care. In their engagements with older boys, shelter workers viewed themselves as powerful gatekeepers of the community; they decided who suffered, how, and with what effects. These understandings determined the demographic makeup of the shelter and how care and resources were distributed among children.[10]

CCI's shelter director, Omar, was responsible for overseeing the children's shelter. He was a tall, burly, and commanding man who spoke fluent English and dressed in a suit and tie every day, indicating that he was the shelter's primary authority figure. His duties entailed hiring aid workers, overseeing shelter activities and finances, and producing administrative reports for Paris headquarters that documented the shelter's daily progress. He was the shelter's primary gatekeeper, because he was the person ultimately responsible for admitting children to the community and discharging them from it. One afternoon, after I asked him how he decided which children could join the shelter, Omar walked me through his entry process. He explained how he administered a two-part examination for every child seeking services at CCI. The first part consisted of formal standardized procedures and included ensuring that the child was under the age of eighteen and homeless. The second part entailed a more informal process and included a one-on-one interview. During the interview, Omar closely observed the child, asked a series of personal questions, and created a file in which the child's life history and healthcare status were recorded. These files were stored in his office at the shelter, in one of several rows of large metal filing cabinets. Aid workers consulted these files in all matters pertaining to a child when problematic situations arose at the shelter. For instance, when a child had an emergency medical condition, engaged in exceptionally problematic behavior, such as fighting or stealing, or was placed on medication, their personal file was pulled and updated with the new data. Children's supposed rehabilitation while at the shelter was tracked through such data. Each personal file captured the child's age, gender, height, weight, appearance at the time of the examination, and physical and emotional health. In addition, the files documented children's former household circumstances, the neighborhoods they were from, how many family members lived in the former household, and the domestic conditions that had led to the child's homelessness or abandonment, according to children's statements.

In explaining the importance of this documented information to me, Omar stressed how he strove to include as much data as possible when compiling new files. He handed me a stack of files, and I flipped through a few of them. The recurring word "divorce" caught my eye—an obvious theme uniting many of the children's stories. I asked Omar how common divorce was among the children's families. Without hesitation, he responded that it was "the main reason" children ended up on the streets. It was also, he believed, one of Egypt's greatest social problems. "People are too quick to divorce and replace a spouse with a new one," he complained. "Then, the children are not wanted by the new spouse. There are a lot of problems between them and then the child leaves or gets kicked out. That is the cause of all this [child homelessness]." As chronicles of children's predicaments and identities, the narratives Omar helped to produce were vivid and dramatic testaments to domestic suffering and social upheaval. Once on paper, these stories became files that situated each child within a network of writing. This writing constructed child subjects and informed disciplinary practices.[11] Together, however, the narratives constituted a body of statistical knowledge about Cairo's streets. Like the data logs mentioned in chapter 2, this information was sent to CCI's Paris headquarters to inform national public health policies and grant applications that would potentially secure more future funding.[12]

Omar stood up, put away the files, and began walking me through his one-on-one interview process. In order to enter the shelter, children had to meet three main criteria. First, he stressed that they had to be visibly *min al shariʿ*, living on the streets. This meant the child had to exhibit the marks of homelessness: an unmistakably thin, frail body, worn-out, dirty clothes, an odor that indicated they were on the streets, and unwashed, matted hair. Omar believed these physical markers of homelessness also revealed inner trauma and vulnerability, associated with loss of family and domestic protection. Next, children also had to perform a degree of submission or passivity to adult authority. If they had an abrasive attitude or seemed uncooperative during the interview, they were denied entry. On the contrary, children who conveyed respect, cooperation, and childlike submission were more likely to be admitted. This factor meant that older or teenage boys, those street children who displayed the highest level of assertiveness, strength, or toughness during the interview, were more likely to be excluded. Ironically, these same masculine characteristics—strength, toughness, and independence—were beneficial to boys on the streets and helped them form successful relationships and money earning outcomes. As Farha Ghannam has shown in an ethnographic study of masculinity in Cairo, strength and toughness constitute attributes of the "respectable man." In Cairo, masculine respectability is bound up with assertiveness and independence, as well as financial productivity and generosity to others. Boys and young men on the streets work hard to achieve these aspects of manhood. They do so in order to earn respect from others, but also to secure their safety on the streets and cultivate a dignified life amidst their economic and social disenfranchisement. Yet in the humanitarian space of CCI's shelter, where submission and passivity mark the deserving child subject and where compassion is distributed through the registers of submission and visible bodily vulnerability, independence and assertiveness worked against street boys.[13] Fearing problems such as violence at the shelter, Omar treated overly independent and assertive street boys with caution.

The third aspect guiding the interview process had to do with whether Omar believed the child would stay at the shelter over the long run. Keeping children off the streets for extended periods of time, offering them vital medical care, and rehabilitating them from the effects of homelessness were the primary goals of the shelter and indicators that the institution had produced successful outcomes. Outcomes were critical nodal points in organizational policy reports. Children who left the shelter, either temporarily or permanently, posed difficulties for aid workers who were tasked with documented children's rehabilitation status, because their health, hygiene, and overall welfare could not be accurately measured or quantified in reports. Boys who left the shelter and returned were considered particularly problematic, because they wavered between two social worlds, one in which they were a dependent "child" living under the care and supervision of shelter aid workers, and the other in which they inhabited the realm of independent "adulthood" on the streets, earning income, smoking, and possibly engaging in sex and drug use.

On the other hand, children who expressed dependency on the shelter and who appeared cooperative during the interview process were likely to be admitted into the shelter. These were the children Omar described as a perfect "fit" for the community. They were also the children who were the youngest, sometimes as young as five years old, and the ones who exhibited the most normative feminized characteristics, such as passivity and submission. As we spoke, Omar elaborated on the differences between these two kinds of children, the deserving and the suspicious street child:

When they first come to me, I make sure they are really *min al shariʿ*. This I can tell just by looking at them, their clothes and face, their hair. Then I talk to them and check to see if they can fit into the community here and get along with others without causing us problems. I only allow in the kids I believe will stay and not run away back to the streets when they feel like it, only to return after some time, begging me to come back in again. This is a big problem we have here, kids coming and going. If I think this will not happen, I let them in.

As this passage makes clear, for Omar being "from the streets" was a status that could be read on the child's body. Hair, face, skin, weight, and clothes all served as material evidence proving that children were homeless. Children also had to be cooperative, dependent, and passive (enough) during the interview. Together, these physical and performative aspects of street-child vulnerability dictated humanitarian inclusion or exclusion. In intimate, daily encounters between workers and children at the shelter, ranging from the entry interview to mealtime, vulnerability was routinely read by aid workers on the child's body. Bodies told stories and narrated histories of suffering and pain. Some children received care and resources as a result of this, while others—typically older boys—were approached with caution and exclusion.

At the other end of this gendered spectrum of visible childhood suffering was girlhood vulnerability. Aid workers typically engaged very young girls as wholly passive and purely innocent sufferers, as the organization's most deserving aid subjects. I witnessed gatekeeping along these lines one afternoon while I was speaking with the shelter's literal gatekeeper, a middle-aged security guard named Mehdi. He was hired from the local neighborhood to monitor the entrance and exit points and ensure that the community remained safe from intruders. Mehdi covered the daytime shift and stood near the main front gate from 9:00 a.m. to approximately 5:00 p.m. each day, keeping a watchful eye on everyone who came in or left the shelter. Because his job was to monitor everyone who entered and departed the premises, Mehdi was the first and last person I spoke with every time I arrived at the shelter. Early on, he had become an important figure in my research. When the children's activities were slow or life at the shelter mundane, I chatted with him about the news, weather, or the latest happenings that day. During one of our extended talks at the shelter's front gate, two young girls we had never encountered before caught our attention as they walked towards the shelter. They approached us swiftly, barefoot, thin arms locked, and skipping, almost playfully. Their dresses were worn-out and their long, matted hair was ruffled by the afternoon wind. Both girls embodied the characteristics of the deserving street child as outlined by Omar. Mehdi briefly glanced at the girls before giving them a wave of the hand and saying, "*Khushu!*" (Enter!). Exhibiting slight annoyance at the brief interruption, Mehdi returned to our talk as if the incident had never occurred.

Given how strict shelter protocol was with respect to entry, I was perplexed as to why he had waved the two unfamiliar girls in without speaking to them or asking any questions. Mehdi laughed, pointed towards the girls, and responded matter-of-factly, "Can't you see, these girls are from the streets and they are beaten [*madrubin*]." For Mehdi, the notion of "beaten" here, as conveyed by the word *madrubin*, framed the girls as beaten up or abused, either by people or by the city itself. In each connotation, the comment referenced girls' bodies as the site of violence. To be "beaten up" in the manner Mehdi conveyed it was to also suffer the additional pain of trauma. Clearly, as he suggested, the girls were suffering enough simply based on their appearance, gender, and extremely young age. His views reaffirmed the ways in which very young girls were seen by workers at CCI as wholly unthreatening and as pure victims. Their gender, age, and vulnerable-looking bodies worked together to arouse immediate humanitarian generosity in Mehdi.

Discretionary judgments about children were made at CCI during lengthy one-on-one interviews like those administered by Omar and through quick, fleeting encounters like that of Mehdi's brief acknowledgment of the two young girls who approached us that afternoon. Whether these encounters were swift or extended, they had lasting effects for children. Aid workers located children along a gendered spectrum that ranged from pure innocence, on the one hand, to suspiciousness, on the other. This spectrum was structured around shared local understandings of victimhood and violence—where young girls were believed to suffer the most on the streets and older boys were thought of as embodying a potential threat—and dictated humanitarian inclusion or exclusion. In turn, flows of care, compassion, and material resources from aid workers to children in daily life at the shelter resulted from such understandings. This was how gender significantly shaped the range of humanitarian possibilities afforded to children at the shelter. But gender also shaped how biomedical experts understood children's trauma and the social effects it could produce if left untreated.

NEGOTIATIONS IN PSYCHIATRIC CARE FOR STREET CHILDREN

Dr. Mona was a native of Cairo and mother of three young children herself. Part-time work with CCI during the days was the ideal job for her; it allowed her to work flexible hours and enjoy quality time with her children in the evenings. Like Dr. Mohamad (see the previous chapter), she had been educated in a respectable Cairo university and spoke fluent English. She was impeccably dressed for work in a dark, professional pant suit, with her hair neatly secured away from her face in a bun. The added touch of a white doctor's coat gave Dr. Mona biomedical authority. To my surprise, however, I realized after speaking with her at length that she was far more critical than I might have supposed of attempts to medicalize street children. In her clinic, she discussed her experiences as a psychiatric care provider at CCI. As she explained, roughly a third of the children at the shelter were receiving psychotropic medication under her supervision. Most of these children, she stressed, were boys whom she considered to be deviant or unstable in ways that threatened themselves or others. For instance, they had started fights with aid workers, intimidated other children, were exceptionally withdrawn, or engaged in acts of misconduct she believed required mood alteration. She diagnosed these children as suffering from "depression," "mood instabilities," and childhood "anxiety disorders." Wanting to probe these medical categorizations further, I asked Dr. Mona why boys at the clinic suffered so frequently from these conditions. She pulled out a large black binder full of papers and vigorously flipped through its many pages. She stopped at a page and pulled out what appeared to be an empty form. Placing it in front of me, she began discussing it in detail. "This is my diagnosis process," she pointed to the top of the page. It was CCI's standard psychiatric examination form, a document that circulated through the organization's international offices. Dr. Mona delved into its importance in guiding her diagnostic practices. It was designed to capture children's emotional status during their first appointment with her.

Bureaucratic practices such as the completion of medical examination forms—conceived by some as rationalized power—were critical to Dr. Mona's work in the clinic. But as many scholars of medical humanitarianism have noted, bureaucracy itself is fraught with human contingencies and a certain degree of guesswork.[14] Moreover, the psychiatric diagnosis is, as we have learned from medical anthropologists, inherently cultural. A medical professional's interpretation, language, and culture shape the psychiatric encounter as well as its outcomes.[15] This became clearly apparent to me when speaking with Dr. Mona about how she completed the form. She spoke about violence on the streets and how Cairo's urban poverty created painful experiences for boys. "Boys suffer from terrible physical violence on the streets, and this causes them emotional pain and trauma," she mentioned with a stern, disconcerted face. "Violence," she continued, "leads to mood instabilities." Each time she treated a boy from CCI in her office, Dr. Mona strove to elicit stories about this street violence, but she emphasized that this was a difficult subject for former street children. Because according to her they were often reluctant to "talk about trauma," she had to recognize its effects on their bodies. She accomplished this by watching patients closely and paying attention to their facial expressions, bodily comportment, and outward physical condition. After probing for signs of "unstable" inner states and visible traces of trauma, she compiled her observations into a story that was written into the examination form. Each form remained in the patient's permanent file in her office and rendered children psychiatric subjects and objects of medical knowledge, of Dr. Mona's medical gaze.

At Dr. Mona's request, I took a long, hard look at an empty form. It was lengthy, over eight pages, and elicited a remarkable amount of writing and what I could only assume was human interpretation. It was typed in English, the standard language of CCI's offices in the Middle East, and consisted of five major sections labeled Personal Data, History, Mental Status, Thoughts, and Results. There were additional subsections for the inclusion of a child's life history, which moved chronologically from Birth and Infancy, to Childhood and Adolescence. Other sections required a deeper analysis of the child's appearance and behavior, with spaces designated for longer entries for descriptions of the child's Mood, Affect, and Speech. The last section, labeled Results, left an entire page free for an extensive handwritten summary of a child's overall emotional health and well-being. According to Cheryl Mattingly, medical charts of this kind reflect a special strategy of medical storytelling. They produce a flat rendering of characters through a process of selective data collection, and capture small moments "here and there" according to an organized chronicle. This medical storytelling keeps the professional's clinical gaze firmly in place.[16]

After putting away the examination forms, Dr. Mona delved into how she spoke with children during their initial medical diagnoses. As she made clear, she always began with a general set of questions designed to comfort her patients and encourage conversation in a "non-threatening" manner. This was important to her because she believed all street children were afraid of adults and were inclined to withhold their true feelings from them. She described how these initial conversations usually unfolded with children: "When I first see them, I just try to start a conversation, like friends. We talk together, and I ask, 'What do you do? How do you see your life? What are your problems and how do you face them? Are you upset about something?' We handle the problem together through behavioral psychotherapy."

After initiating a conversation in this manner, Dr. Mona then attempted to elicit stories from boy patients about their former drug use and smoking practices. She understood how widespread smoking and drugs were among street children and felt strongly about getting children "clean." She believed drug use and smoking had a direct correlation to trauma, and that children who engaged in these practices would continue to experience "inner disorders" and "behavior problems." It was difficult for her, however, to convince boy patients to stop these practices. Often, she would gently and indirectly suggest to boys that they quit, rather than demand they do so, before offering them medication as the solution to their suffering: "I advise him, but indirectly, for example, about drug use and smoking. I encourage them to do the best for themselves and get the problem out from inside so that I can show them how to solve it. Then I ask, "What do you think [about my prescribing] you something?'"

Dr. Mona's diagnosis process was dialogical, one in which she conversed with children and advised them on how to "get their problems out from the inside." She strove to help children release their inner thoughts and get them out into the open so that they could become the object of therapeutic intervention. She believed that boys were mutually responsible for this process, that they should invest in their own rehabilitation and contribute to their own emotional healing. As her comments made clear, she emphasized this dialogical approach by asking children how they felt about her prescribing medication for them.

Boys clearly had a degree of agency during their psychiatric appointments with Dr. Mona. But sometimes this agency restricted her care practices and resembled biomedical resistance. In speaking to me about medication, Dr. Mona described how boys had a capacity to comply or resist her prescriptions, and this affected her medical practice. She would most often prescribe medication when she was able to clearly "see" inner suffering or trauma surface during the psychiatric diagnosis process. For instance, as she explained, a boy's energy at the time of the examination could determine whether or not she prescribed him medication. As she understood it, children who had lived on the streets, like those served by CCI, were unable to trust or openly speak to adult authority figures. This was because of their experiences with adult oppression, either in their former households or from the police on the streets. Therefore, when a child appeared sluggish, lethargic, uncooperative during therapy, or apathetic, he was more likely to be put on a regimen of mood stabilizers. Children's manner of speech and overall responsiveness also strongly influenced whether or not they were put on medication. Dr. Mona further elaborated on the importance of seeing these visible signs of disorder first, before prescribing medication: "I must observe his affect and his mood, and his facial expressions, and I ask him directly, 'How do you see life?' But I don't just listen to what they say. I must look at their bodies and watch their gestures. I have to do a lot of investigating and guessing. Then I try to put it all together, like pieces in a puzzle."

Although she recognized that girls experienced severe forms of gendered violence and adult oppression on the streets as well, Dr. Mona believed boys suffered disproportionately from biological mood instabilities and hyperactivity as a result of their experiences on the streets. That, she warned, could lead to violence in and beyond the street children's shelter. For her, medication constituted a relatively safe and humane solution to their potentially threatening suffering. We talked at length about the ways in which medication targeted aggression. Drugs, she asserted, "help control aggression and violence," and they substantially increased a boy's ability to listen to and take adult advice. For her boy patients, she typically prescribed antidepressants belonging to the Carbamazepine group of anticonvulsants. In particular, she preferred the cheap and readily available drug sold under the trade name Tegretol and believed it was an ideal drug for street-child patients.[17] It was provided by CCI at her request, and produced minimal side effects in treating mood disorders. Dr. Mona reiterated, however, that resistance to her pharmaceutical prescriptions was common among the boys she treated at CCI. When she encountered resistance, either during therapy sessions or towards her suggested pharmaceutical regimens, she worked hard to convince her patients that psychiatry had value, and psychotropic medication could help. Like other medical professionals, she had to coax some of her patients into accepting certain healthcare regimens.[18]

As we spoke further, Dr. Mona's contradictory views about the work CCI was doing with street children began to surface. Despite her belief that psycho-pharmaceutical therapy was a legitimate intervention for street-child trauma and a means towards emotional rehabilitation for boys with behavior problems, she still shared feelings of apprehension about it and doubted the long-term efficacy of her care. Moreover, she understood that her young patients practiced medical noncompliance and frequently resisted her advice during talk therapy, just as they resisted other authority figures at CCI. Some of her boy patients, for example, ran away from the shelter to work on the streets when they believed it was best for them to do so, only to return when they desired. When they returned, they reengaged with their mandatory pharmaceutical regimen only because they had to, but they often abruptly stopped treatment once they left again. Because of this, Dr. Mona felt it was crucial to prescribe drugs that did not cause serious side effects in the event treatment was abruptly terminated. Tegretol, according to her, fit that requirement perfectly. She described it as a "mild" and relatively safe medication for children—a good, if not perfect, solution to boys' behavioral disorders.

Global health policy continues to promote a singular biomedical approach to human suffering in the global south, whether that suffering is a result of war, poverty, or natural disasters. Yet local medical aid experts like Dr. Mona grapple with the unresolvable contradictions inherent in their work, the discord between standardized policy and messy local realities. As a humanitarian psychiatrist, Dr. Mona prescribed medication for street children, but she believed the practice had ambiguous effects, because it did not alter the long-term conditions children were living in and because the course of her treatment could be disrupted due to children's practices. In our conversations about street children's conditions, Dr. Mona always shifted the discussion away from medicine and towards Egyptian politics and the widespread economic struggles she was observing around her. She frequently and passionately complained about social transformations she had witnessed over the past two decades, particularly rising food costs. She identified political corruption as the cause of rising poverty rates in Cairo and, in turn, higher rates of child homelessness. Rejecting the belief that medicalization was the magic bullet that would solve street children's problems, Dr. Mona ultimately believed that political and economic solutions, not humanitarian interventions or psychiatry, were urgently needed to address the street-child crisis the country was facing.

Perhaps more than other aid worker I spoke with, Dr. Mona described how difficult street life was for homeless boys. She understood their need to make money and was aware of the scale of violence they encountered from the police and other boys on the streets. After working for CCI delivering psychiatric care for years, she had come to realize that there were forces beyond her control that caused boys to distrust and resist her care. Dr. Mona navigated these tensions as best she could by recognizing boys' economic and political demands, and by engaging boys as active agents during psychotherapy sessions. She strove to rehabilitate boys psychiatrically, while also accommodating them by prescribing "safer" medications when she knew they would reject or disrupt their pharmaceutical regimens. Boys' preferences and potential for noncompliance deeply influenced her medical care. Like Dr. Mohamad in chapter two, she was aware of the limits of her medical authority with aid recipients.

Moving beyond Dr. Mona's clinic, psychiatry played into boys' everyday lives at the shelter in ambiguous ways, sometimes altering their experiences and at others barely affecting their health, daily practices, or relationships. Psychiatry's aim was to rehabilitate children emotionally, to restore hope for boys, but at CCI it was also a source of conflict for boys. A look at how Mahmud negotiated psychiatric care and medication in his daily life, as merely one aspect of his complex social world, will help shed further light on the ways in which that care was productive yet limiting for boys themselves.

THE RECIPIENT OF CHILD PSYCHIATRIC CARE: MAHMUD

After I accompanied him to his therapy session in Dr. Mona's office, Mahmud admitted to me that afternoon when we returned to the shelter that he never enjoyed psychiatric appointments. They seemed to be a minor factor in his life, an interruption, a visit he had to make once a month. Regardless, they produced a negative reaction from him. Watching him in the clinic, it appeared as if he was simply going through the motions. For Mahmud, psycho-pharmaceuticalization represented a loss of his freedom and an affront to his personal agency. It did not represent a form of restorative, compassionate care, at least not in the manner that CCI policy and to some extent Dr. Mona had hoped that it would be. But Mahmud also did not resemble the figure of the street child as it was described in CCI discourse. He actively chose to work on the streets, and once there moved between the streets, humanitarian spaces, and his former household. It was important for him to assert his masculine independence in each of these spaces, which entailed making money and resisting adult authority figures who attempted to control him.

At fourteen, Mahmud was the oldest boy living at the CCI shelter. Towering over the other children, he was also the tallest, and visibly most adult-like of the group. He was one of the first children serviced by the shelter, having lived there on and off for over four years by the time I arrived in 2008. Workers held a special reverence for Mahmud because of his senior status with other children. He was viewed as possessing deep institutional knowledge and approached as capable of some adult tasks, such as carrying large, heavy platters during mealtime. Workers relied on him in ways that marked him as a special elder among the other children. As Sally explained it to me during my early months at the shelter, Mahmud had practically grown up at CCI and was, therefore, a child of the organization. This special status became evident to me early on in my research when I heard her refer to him as a "son of CCI" (*ibn CCI*).

On most days, Mahmud just wanted to speak to me about his passion for being on his own and finding full-time work outside the shelter. He aspired to a skill that would earn him a stable salary and a respectable life. For instance, he stressed to me how much he loved learning about *kahraba* (electricity) at the shelter, and desired to understand computers and work on them. Mastering a technical skill such as electricity or computers would, he believed, enable him to achieve his ultimate goal of becoming a productive adult and employed professional worker.

Mahmud hailed from the low-income neighborhood of Faisal, just slightly west of Giza. He had been ten years old when he left home to work on the streets near the Pyramids. Other kids on the streets mentioned a new place for children called CCI, a welcoming and "good" place to be (*makan kuwayis*). His short yet eventful life history mirrored that of many other children at CCI. His nuclear family had broken apart because of a healthcare crisis and intensifying urban poverty. His mother had died when he was eight. His father, an on-and-off truck driver, never remarried, and his older siblings—two brothers and a sister—struggled to meet the household's demands, which included a rising cost of living. In their one-bedroom apartment, Mahmud felt particularly disempowered. As the youngest male, he suffered physical abuse and intimidation by his father and older brother. But this abuse was not the primary factor that compelled him to leave his home for the streets. It was a conflict related to economic demands associated with public schooling, demands his father either could not or refused to meet.

This is how Mahmud described this life-transformative moment to me: one day, he asked his father to take care of some important administrative work and school fees at his public school. His father refused and kept brushing off the request. "He just wouldn't do it, he kept ignoring me," Mahmud explained, reflecting on that momentous day. Because of this neglect, Mahmud was kicked out of school, forbidden to return. He viewed this exclusion as a major setback, an obstacle in his life. In theory, public education is free to all Egyptians, but in practice attendance requires bribes be paid to teachers and administrators. Most families struggle to meet these demands, while others must hire private tutors for children in order to supplement sub-par lessons given by overworked and underpaid public schoolteachers. Increasingly, low-income families struggle to meet these perpetually rising informal costs attached to public education. Disempowered at home and now excluded from school, lacking an alternative system of social support, Mahmud believed, at the age of ten, that the streets were a better, more productive, place for him to be.

On the streets, Mahmud joined a network of boys ranging in age from five to nineteen. They traveled together in and out of busy city neighborhoods and the tourist zone around the Pyramids. Although he was often subjected to street fights with other children and endured police harassment, Mahmud talked about this environment and the work on the streets as being immensely profitable, earning him sometimes nearly twenty Egyptian pounds a day, approximately US$4.50 at the time of this research. Mahmud had a system in place for handling his cash. He saved half of the day's income and allocated the other half to that day's immediate expenses, which typically included cheap street food, cigarettes, hot tea, and sodas supplied by local street vendors.

Mahmud was not only working for his own survival and sense of independence on the streets however. He periodically delivered a portion of his saved income to his younger sister in his former household in Faisal. She was the only person he felt obligated to visit and support financially after his departure from home. Realizing the extent to which poverty governed her life, Mahmud felt responsible for his sister. This sense of responsibility stemmed from normative models of masculinity in Cairo. As an older brother, Mahmud spoke about his sister in terms of his fear for her, his need to protect her, specifically from immoral sexual acts that she could possibly commit due to her and the family's impoverishment. As he stated it, he didn't want her to "do something shameful for money" and thereby tarnish his reputation or his family's reputation in their tight-knit neighborhood.

According to CCI policy, Mahmud was a homeless, dependent, traumatized street child. But his day-to-day practices indicate that he was also a gendered subject who had desires, obligations, and affective ties to home. He was also a caregiver to a younger sister who was not considered "homeless" in CCI aid policy but who nonetheless suffered from poverty and forms of violence that global aid organizations would consider child rights abuses. While she remained outside of CCI's humanitarian reach, Mahmud refused to be completely governed by it.

At the shelter, I first learned Mahmud was consuming psycho-pharmaceuticals when I caught a glimpse of him swallowing a pill after lunch one afternoon in the shelter's courtyard. Hany, who served as a part-time social worker for the children, handed Mahmud a white paper cup containing a Tegratol tablet, with water to wash it down. He then stood by Mahmud, paternalistically, to supervise the consumption and ensure Mahmud had swallowed the medication. As the pill went down with a quick swig of bottled water, Hany gently placed a hand on Mahmud's shoulder, as if to say he had done well, and walked away. During his sessions with Dr. Mona, the effects Tegratol had on Mahmud were carefully monitored. She reassured him that the medication was working and thus necessary. In talk therapy sessions, Mahmud spoke to Dr. Mona about his former household in Faisal, his time on the streets, and difficulties he was experiencing at the shelter. Dr. Mona would then encourage him to remain at the shelter and not to run away. She urged him to stick to his pharmaceutical regimen, because it was good for him. It was, she stressed in therapy sessions, part of the emotional rehabilitation process and critical if he were to achieve optimum mental health, inner stability.

Just as in other studies that have documented children's resistance to psychiatric medication, I too discovered that Mahmud viewed Tegratol as a form of social control.[19] He approached this medication just like other interventions he received at the shelter, as an oppressive, governing practice that he did not want to submit to. When he spoke to me about being placed on medication and having to visit Dr. Mona, he confessed that he did not appreciate it when people told him what to do and "governed" him (*hakamu fiya*). At the shelter, he felt as if his freedom (*huriya*) was increasing being lost. All the rules and hierarchies between adults and children seemed to suffocate him, as they had in his former household. On the contrary, the streets represented a form of emancipation for him, even if they posed the constant threat of violence and insecurity. For these reasons, he ran away from the shelter often, for anywhere between a week to several months. During these departures, he returned to making money on the streets and reconnected with his old friends. He checked up on his sister and gave her some cash, and this allowed him to meet his gendered obligations while regaining a sense of masculine independence. Also, while on the streets, he stopped taking Tegratol and, in an act that directly challenged CCI's efforts to produce biomedically healthy street children, he started smoking cigarettes again.

Life on the streets was difficult for Mahmud, sometimes because it was lonely and at others because it was not safe or particularly economically productive. For these reasons, he returned to the shelter, reunited with friends there, and enjoyed a necessary respite from street life, even if, as a result, it meant a loss of his personal freedom. Aid workers at the shelter made exceptions for Mahmud because of his deep ties to the organization and his reputation as a well-known member of the community when he was there. Because of his age status, and the affection workers held for him, he was granted special reentry privileges. His inevitable sojourns away from the shelter were tolerated by aid workers, albeit with exasperation.

Mahmud's practice of leaving the shelter to work on the streets was not uncommon among the children at CCI. Nada, described in chapter 1, and many other children at the shelter left from time to time to work on the streets, return home, or receive aid from other institutions. For aid workers, children's mobility was an obstinate problem. It was considered antithetical to the goals of the street-child shelter. But it nonetheless remained a significant aspect of street children's experiences there.

Mahmud negotiated his masculinity and desire for independence alongside his status as a "traumatized" child and global aid recipient at CCI. Psychiatry, talk therapy, and psycho-pharmaceuticals did not seem directly harmful to Mahmud as he navigated multiple social spaces and identities—between home, shelter, and the streets—but they also did not seem to achieve their intended goals either—which was to stabilize Mahmud's moods and get him to remain at the shelter under the watchful eyes of adult aid workers. Psychiatry, like other medical aid interventions at CCI, did not address Mahmud's need for money, his desire to feel like a man, or his obligation to care for his younger sister, a practice that would help ensure his family's reputation remained positive in the eyes of their community. For him, compulsory talk therapy and psycho-pharmaceuticals represented a complex site of struggle, with CCI's shelter resembling a space of care as well as a governing institution. CCI was one home among others for Mahmud. As Tobias Hecht notes in writing about street children in Brazil who were similarly institutionalized, the shelter, replete with free psychiatric care, was far from a solution to his homelessness. It was simply "an integral part of the street life experience."[20]

Mahmud displayed extraordinary resilience as a decision-making, gendered subject on the streets and as a recipient of CCI's shelter, but the implications of his experiences with global psychiatric care remain troubling in light of how medication functions in local contexts. Through practices defined by CCI as emotional care, as compassionate intervention, aid workers further marginalized him as pathologized and as a "problem," a potentially violent masculine subject. As a result, care took the form of pharmaceutical intervention, mood stabilization, and behavioral normalization. Within the complex assemblages of care that Mahmud experienced at CCI, between the shelter and Dr. Mona's clinic, aid workers tethered his inner state and gender to notions of a better, more secure future society. In this way, humanitarian psychiatry at CCI produced paradoxical effects for Mahmud, effects that concretized his status as a vulnerable child yet potentially dangerous male subject.

Chapter 4

DO MUSLIM VILLAGE GIRLS NEED SAVING?

ONE DAY IN CAIRO, OVER COFFEE IN A CROWDED DOWNTOWN CAFÉ, Philippe, a French global aid worker, told me that the Muslim village girl was global aid's "ultimate victim, the best victim."[1] At the time, Philippe was directing the International Village Girl Project (IVGP; the name has been changed to protect anonymity), a major global youth initiative in the Middle East and North Africa focused on girls living in "traditional" rural settings. Between sips of frothy cappuccino, he explained that village girls evoked "the most compassion" from powerful donors and policy-makers working for international aid institutions, thus generating the most funds. I asked Philippe what it meant for him, as the director of a village girl youth project, to recognize the "Muslim village girl" as a salient and capacious category in aid. Philippe was candid in his response. He elaborated how the Muslim village girl appeared exceptionally "savable" to aid experts because, like the figure of the child, she was an unquestionably innocent, agentless sufferer. But she was different from the child. Her adolescent age status, gender, and Muslim identity rendered her a sufferer in multiple and intersecting ways. She was the victim of poverty but also of gendered violence and religious fundamentalism. In global aid policy, these multiple layers of vulnerability were articulated as legitimizing features of intervention for village girls; they compelled distant populations to act on their behalf.

Philippe was in his early thirties. For several years prior to our interview, he had lived in North Africa and the Middle East promoting global humanitarian

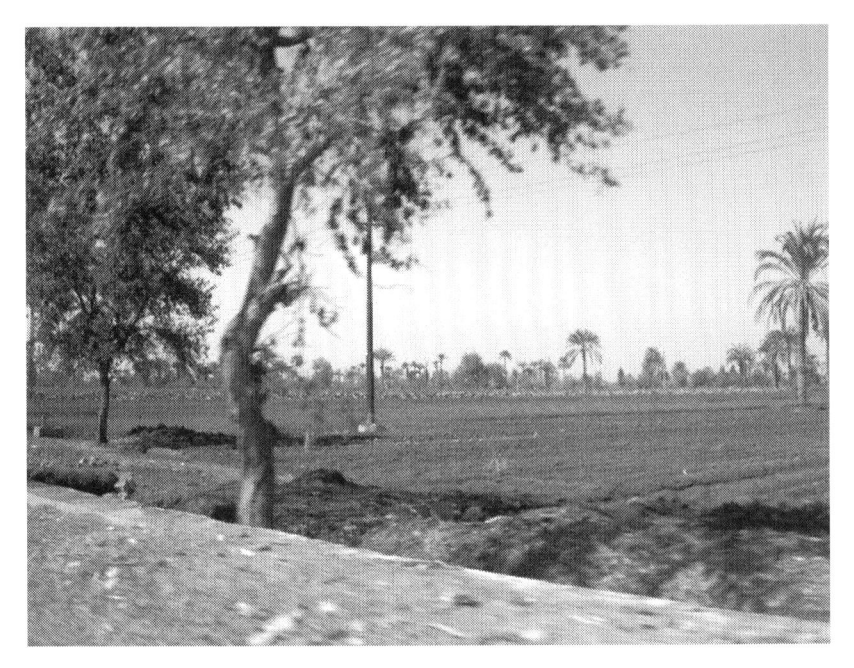

FIGURE 5. Agricultural land in Beni Suef, 2008. Photograph by the author.

and development initiatives focused on vulnerable girls. His extended time in the field and experiences producing aid policy as an administrator taught him that village girls were, in his words, "the best" victims because they drove entire international moral economies of aid.[2] Who could contest their suffering, their inherent victimhood, or their desperate need for assistance from the global north, he proclaimed with an undertone of sarcasm, as they navigated poverty and strict patriarchal norms? According to Philippe, these were the cultural and affective registers attached to the Muslim village girl category in global aid policy.

These registers of Muslim village girl suffering are not only present in global aid policy. They also frame depictions in popular culture, literature, and media about the Middle East and North Africa. In 2010, for example, *I am Nujood, Age 10 and Divorced*, a gripping book recounting the life history of a ten-year-old Yemeni village girl, was published in English by Three Rivers Press.[3] It targeted a wide international readership and was crafted to invoke compassion for village girls living in Muslim societies, telling how Nujood endured child marriage in Yemen, a place the co-author, Delphine Minoui, describes as an, "extraordinary and turbulent

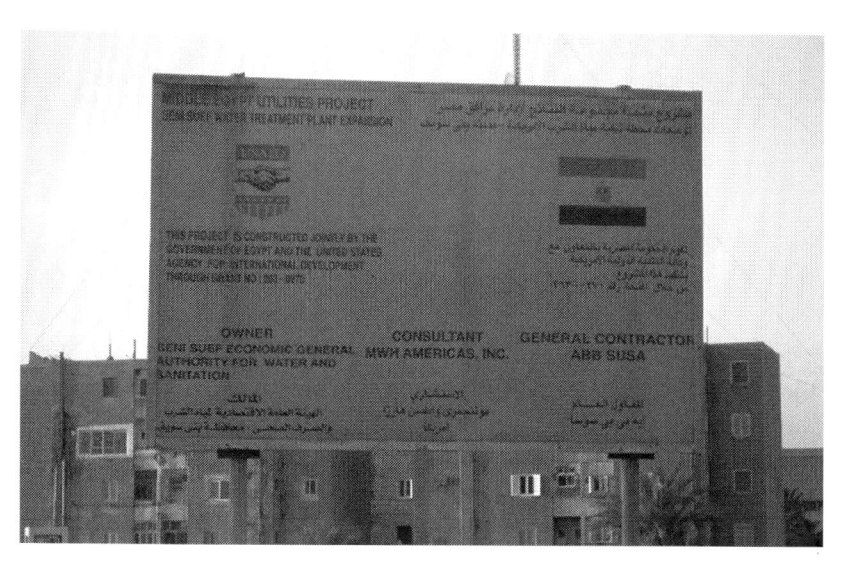

FIGURE 6. A sign upon entry into Beni Suef reflects the strong presence of USAID, 2008. Photograph by the author.

country."⁴ Early on in the book, we are introduced to Nujood's gentle, childlike face and veiled hair, which also grace the book's front cover. Minoui introduces Nujood using universal language about the child, mirroring international children's rights discourse, writing, "A tiny wisp of a thing, Nujood is neither queen nor princess. She is a normal girl with parents and plenty of brothers and sisters. Like all children her age, she loves to play hide-and-seek and adores chocolate."⁵

Painted as an innocent victim of poverty, patriarchal oppression, and Islamic extremism, Nujood is eventually granted a divorce from a husband three times her age. Her liberation is brought about by an urban, middle-class professional, a woman lawyer whose job it is to emancipate vulnerable girls. As the book poignantly makes clear, upon her divorce, Nujood gained her girlhood back and was freed from the bonds of marriage, able to enjoy her dreams of going to school, foster friendships, and play with toys. *Glamour* magazine named Nujood Woman of the Year, and Hillary Clinton enthusiastically endorsed the book, calling Nujood her "hero" and one of the "greatest women" she had ever seen. Reflecting what Partha Chatterjee termed an "effervescent sympathy for the oppressed," Nujood's story had a powerful appeal among readers in the United States and Western Europe.⁶ This same appeal has recently propelled a wide range of global humanitarian aid initiatives focused exclusively on "Third World girls," including the popular

UN-backed Girl Up campaign. Driven by a mixture of child rights, biomedical, and liberal feminist logics, these campaigns focus on the intersecting problems of economic rural underdevelopment and gender violence as experienced by out-of-school adolescent girls.

This chapter is concerned with one such humanitarian initiative as it took place in the southern Egyptian governorate of Beni Suef. While there in 2008, I conducted ethnographic research on the IVGP. As we have seen in the case of other contemporary global aid initiatives designed to liberate local women from gender oppression in the Middle East, IVGP policy deployed a set of othering discourses about girlhood, villages, Islam, and culture in order to further its aims and expand the initiative. Present in popular media like *I am Nujood*, these discourses reproduced an imaginary cultural divide between East and West, as well as hierarchical relations between cities and villages, and local men, women, boys, and girls.[7] Such humanitarian campaigns end up speaking *for* village girls, while situating global aid workers in positions of power vis-à-vis village families and communities. Moving beyond the aid policy that fails to address the problem of rural poverty, this chapter pays close attention to the perspectives of village girls. It also focuses on the identities of aid workers, their opinions about the project, and the ways in which they enacted it in offices and villages. In doing so, this chapter offers a deeper and more critical look into how a global village girl campaign took hold in Egypt with paradoxical effects, and through encounters between workers, girl recipients, and their families.

In my interviews with the aid workers who implemented the IVGP, I found that village girls often became the contested ground through which broader social and political claims were advanced. In speaking with girls who participated in the IVGP, I got a sense of how they simultaneously enjoyed the project *and* managed it as one additional obligation in their duty-filled lives. As I dug deeper into these intersecting humanitarian contradictions, I analyzed the aid policy in depth and found that it drew on global health and rights paradigms as well as preexisting stereotypes about Islam, villages, and gender relations in the Middle East. In addition, it rarely represented the desires and social lives of girls to their fullest. Like most humanitarian projects that are implemented in rural contexts, the IVGP did not meet its formally stated aims, nor did it even attempt to transform the structural conditions that kept adolescent girls out of formal schools in Egypt. It did, however, set into motion a range of processes, challenges, and negotiations for girls, their families, and aid workers that present a more nuanced picture of global girl-centered humanitarianism than popular media or policy typically captures. More importantly, the IVGP generated substantial funding from international donor institutions. This funding buttressed the project's expansion and reproduced its work.

In many ways, in her book, Nujood appeared strikingly similar to the village girls I met in Beni Suef. She donned similar modest dress—a head scarf and long robe—and had ambitions to go to school and get a job. She conveyed a similar sense of imaginative adventure and optimism about her future. However, the girls I interviewed in Beni Suef had more expansive ideas about what girlhood meant to them. They shared desires about marriage and engaged in kinship practices that challenged global aid representations of village girl passivity and suffering. Perhaps Nujood had more diverse ideas about girlhood as well. If she did, however, those ideas remain mediated/or eclipsed by the author who conveyed her story to the world. To me it appeared as if the girls in Beni Suef had stakes in the IVGP that were at clear odds with those of global aid policy-makers. Without discounting or neglecting the very real ways in which girls in villages throughout the Middle East and North Africa actually do suffer, this chapter probes the appeal and institutional power the figure of the Muslim village girl wields within global medical aid.

LEGACIES OF GENDERED ORIENTALISM

Before I delve into the defining features of the IVGP, it is critical to note that global initiatives targeting adolescent girls in rural contexts have not emerged in a vacuum.[8] These campaigns follow a longer history of international humanitarian and human rights initiatives focused on the plight of Third World adult women. As we have seen for centuries, the desire to save Muslim women from local men and governments follows a legacy of Western colonial intervention in the Middle East. Drawing on Edward Said's foundational work *Orientalism*, as well as in-depth ethnographic research with Egyptian women for decades, Lila Abu-Lughod discusses this impulse as a form of "gendered orientalism." In an impactful book on transnational feminism titled *Do Muslim Women Need Saving?* Abu-Lughod contests universalized claims, often made by global human rights experts, that Egyptian women need emancipation from gendered and religious oppression. In interviews with Egyptian women, Abu-Lughod discovered that it was not so much gender or religious oppression that women believed they needed liberation from. Rather, it was global economic policies, a Western-backed authoritarian government, and ongoing systemic poverty that were the primary causes of their suffering.

Underneath its rhetoric of salvation, however, gendered orientalism is incredibly powerful, particularly with respect to foreign policy in the Middle East. According to Abu-Lughod, it has fueled an imaginary separation between the West and Islam and has, for decades, buttressed a growing number of transnational humanitarian governing initiatives in the region.[9] Along with furthering an orientalist perspective about the entire Middle East, gendered orientalism, conveyed through harrowing stories about oppression and liberation like *I am Nujood*, performs cultural and racial work in the realm of global aid and humanitarianism. It reinforces a set of discourses about Islam and poverty, pinning ideas of tradition (the rural) and modernization (the urban) against each other.[10] As Said explicated in his concept of orientalism, what one pole is (read modern, free, and urban), the other cannot be (backward, oppressed, and rural). Nujood, it is important to stress, was emancipated from her forced marriage not by women in her own community but by an urban professional, a woman lawyer, who intervened on her behalf and disrupted traditional village practices, despite the fierce opposition she faced.

Transnational feminist scholars have criticized global interventions in the name of gender liberation—from military campaigns to development projects—for decades now because they have found that such interventions reproduce ethnocentric and racist views about Muslim women and their societies. In addition, the interventions assume a position of First World dominance over the Third World, and advance "imperial feminist" agendas—a form of feminism that assumes that white Western women bear the inherent burden of liberating women around the world. As transnational feminists have argued, imperial feminism elides various intersections of class, nation, ethnicity, and sexuality in experiences of oppression and keeps global racial hierarchies intact.[11] The most radical work produced by transnational feminist scholars has even forced us to rethink many of the underlying presuppositions driving liberal feminist thought, such as the concepts of "individual autonomy," "self-actualization," and "freedom."[12] These categories, they contend, are culturally and historically specific, and have spread to regions like the Middle East through colonial processes, military campaigns, and neoliberal economic relations.

NEITHER A CHILD NOR AN ADULT: THE GIRL AS TRANQUILIZING OBJECT

Even as they draw on this legacy of gendered orientalism, girl-centered global humanitarian aid campaigns have their own distinct features and social effects. These differences warrant new questions around who needs saving, why, and from whom. According to Philippe, the Muslim village girl, like the street child in Cairo, is approached as an apolitical sufferer. In formal global aid policy, she is constructed as a gendered sufferer and a biological girl with universalized female features. Biology and her unmarried liminal social status mark her as different from adult Muslim women and *more* vulnerable. Philippe understood the affective force attached to this biological vulnerability in policy, its power to inspire action. He articulated a heady critique of how global aid organizations increasingly use adolescent girlhood to secure grants and generate work. He believed the deployment of the village girl category in policy was suspicious, but at the same time, he felt it was necessary to deploy the category in order to maintain positive aid outcomes and expand initiatives in places like rural Egypt. Interestingly, he seemed to live with this irreconcilable contradiction even if it caused him unease and moments of critical self-reflection, as it had during our interview.

In IVGP reports, grants, and statistics, the lives of village girls were framed by the intersecting registers of bodily and economic oppression. Terms such as, "confinement in the home, lack of education, underdevelopment, exposure to child marriage, exposure to violent traditional practices, and perpetual poverty," were used to describe their daily conditions. The policy isolated girls for intervention, labeling them a "forgotten class," a silenced group within their own households and society. The aid discourses further highlighted the girl body, with its budding sexuality, as requiring compassion and intervention. The IVGP claimed that puberty itself exposed these girls to more gender-based violence than women, implicitly marking boys and men as sources of that violence. Moving beyond "womanhood" as the site of global intervention, here "girlhood," and particularly the developing biological female body, signaled a life phase that exposed girls to specific social conditions and forms of oppression. As the policy expressed it, puberty in Egyptian villages placed girls in dangerous liminal social status, one that children, boys, or adult women did not occupy. The aid policy emphasized how puberty differed for girls in Egyptian rural contexts. Rather than constituting a phase in the human life cycle marked by greater personal freedoms, puberty in Egyptian villages restricted girl mobility. This was because, as the policy stated, adolescent girls were viewed as reproductive yet unmarried subjects in their communities. This status exposed them to practices such as domestic labor and early (child) marriage, two "child rights abuses" the IVGP strove to eradicate in village contexts.

I find Chandra Mohanty's analysis of the Third World woman in development aid particularly useful in thinking about how the figure of the Muslim village girl has emerged as the quintessential humanitarian object in aid policy recently. In an article titled "Under Western Eyes: Feminist Scholarship and Colonial Discourses," Mohanty claims that international development gains legitimacy around notions of Third World women's dehistoricization and naturalized subordination.[13] Try as they may, agentless local women, as they are depicted in development aid policy, can never rise above their object-status.[14] However, IVGP policy suggests that it is not only gendered vulnerability that gives Muslim village girls a similar object-status, making them the ultimate, agentless victims of a dangerous mixture of patriarchy and poverty. It is also what Liisa Malkki calls the "tranquilizing conventions" attached to humanitarian images of the child.[15] When it comes to village girls, these conventions include descriptions of girls' perceived innocence, their basic human goodness, their developing apolitical bodies, and how they are believed to embody hope for the future developing nation. These conventions have "tranquilizing" effects in aid industries because they espouse an unparalleled level of compassion and action on behalf of girl recipients. As Malkki has outlined for the case of children in dominant Christian images of the human, such charismatic figurations of the suffering young serve to promote global aid in undeveloped countries for the ultimate aims of fund-raising and civilizing entire local populations.[16]

THE IVGP'S GOALS AND BROADER IMPLICATIONS

The IVGP was launched in Egyptian villages in 2001 by a consortium of large-scale international aid organizations, of which CCI was one. Each aid organization had headquarters based in Western Europe or the United States, and operated with established offices in Cairo. In their Cairo offices, highly trained aid workers and administrators collaborated, exchanged knowledge, and formed networks in order to successfully advance the project across southern Egypt. In 2007, I was deep in my internship work at CCI, but chose to work as an unpaid intern in the offices of the United States Development Initiative (USDI) because it was responsible for spearheading and directing the IVGP across Egypt. As such, it served as the ideal research site for questions around global medical aid for village girls.

USDI successfully implemented the IVGP with major funding from the Egyptian state, ExxonMobil, the Ford Foundation, Nike, and the Dutch embassy. In years subsequent to its implementation, it generated a steady influx of grant money, which helped expand the project across rural Egypt. By 2007, approximately six years into its expansion, the IVGP received a follow-up grant of over US$1.8 million to serve around two thousand village girls in two rural Egyptian governorates. With nearly 30 percent of Egypt's population falling below the national poverty line at the time of this research, this represented substantial funding.[17] It signaled the extent to which village girl humanitarian causes had gained traction in Egypt and were remarkably successful at galvanizing support from donors.

Aid experts at USDI helped to craft vivid descriptions of village girls in IVGP policy and grant proposals that evoked compassion especially from urban populations. This discourse presented village girls as radically other, as rural subjects, but also familiar, in that they resembled universalized, middle-class adolescents, or global "youth." Girls were described as having growing vulnerable bodies, a desire to play, learn, socialize with friends, and be "free" (presumably from adult supervision and traditions). One of the first things I learned about the IVGP from aid experts I interviewed was that it was an unprecedented step "forward" in Egyptian history precisely because it targeted a previously overlooked yet extremely vulnerable recipient population. For these aid workers, their focus on adolescent village girls was a source of immense pride. Some complained that the country was turning towards increased public religious conservatism and lauded the project's swift expansion as countering these broad social and political trends. After all, the project aimed to "empower" and "uplift" out-of-school village girls by educating them through a series of classes designed around "life skills." These skills included but were not limited to basic literacy, women's rights, sports and fitness, and adolescent health. Aid workers believed these objectives reinforced girls' access to their legally established rights—the right to education, health, and personal agency. According to one published report, the IVGP intended to accomplish these goals by "intervening into traditional communities," where girls lacked educational opportunities and physical mobility.

The life-skill classes were taught by low-level aid workers who were from the village where the project was operative, and who worked in local youth centers that were chosen for their close proximity to girls' families. Proximity ensured attendance, since it added incentive for those parents who feared the project would take girls too far away from home. Out-of-school girls between the ages of ten and sixteen were chosen to participate. They typically met in groups of twenty to twenty-five, up to four times a week in three-hour sessions. Sometimes older teenage girls who had graduated from previous installments of the project helped run these classes. Given the respectable title of "mentor," these seasoned veteran recipients were tasked with assisting new girls as they transitioned from domestic spaces to the public, and often male-dominated, space of youth centers.

While its primary stated goal was to arm out-of-school village girls with new skills centered on health and rights, the IVGP also strove to reconfigure what it meant to be a girl (*bint*) through the promotion of what I call a global youth habitus—a set of cultivated, embodied habits centered on adolescent hygiene, health, and mobility. Exercising, eating breakfast, socializing with peers, taking showers, and playing sports were among the habits promoted through the project. In IVGP policy as well as in my conversations with USDI workers, these habits signaled the adoption of a universal youthfulness reflecting personal autonomy, emancipation, and freedom. The policy asserted that if these goals were achieved, village girls would enjoy a healthy, normative youth and eventually help lift their villages out of stagnant underdevelopment and traditionalism. The notion that villages would one day "catch up" with cities through global interventions focused on girls was a common theme in the policy.

With its emphasis on futurity and hope as embodied in aid recipients, the IVGP resembled previous state-sanctioned international development projects in Egypt. These projects promoted development through the construction of a new, self-governing self, a modern national citizen. During the early nineteenth century and up to the twentieth century, for example, the state, along with social reformers and European governing bodies, aimed to shape the health and bodily practices of adult villagers in Egypt. Population control policies were put in place with the dual intention of governing reproduction and decreasing population growth. While these policies targeted the intersecting problems of overpopulation and rural poverty, they also advanced the construction of a modern national subjectivity, a new "healthy body." The idea was that new subjects should regulate their individual fertility practices, and new bodies should be autonomous and rights-bearing, in line with global development standards.[18]

While the IVGP shared some of these development goals, it differed from past initiatives by hinging its appeal on the perceived innocence and victimhood of adolescent girls, especially with respect to their vulnerable and growing bodies. Youth around the world, the policy asserted, shared the same desires. They craved freedom from authority figures and harbored a natural desire for sports, fun, and friends. Moreover, they shared a general curiosity about their developing sexuality. Traditional practices in villages, policy suggested, denied girls these natural, universal desires, subjecting them to conservative values and gendered violence. By defining villages as "traditional" spaces, IVGP experts implicitly marked cities as modern spaces devoid of such practices.[19] And while it sought to eradicate "child rights abuses" in villages by instilling rights, the IVGP also strove to reconfigure the biological and social experience of "youth" itself for girls.

MORALITY, SPACE, AND THE CONSTRUCTION OF A NEW GIRL SELF

Another key theme in the policy was morality, which was described as an essential feature of rights for girls and promoted accordingly. The act of emancipating village girls from the conditions in which they lived was framed as morally correct and necessary if girls were to achieve rights. In addition, girl emancipation would be economically and socially productive for villages, the nation, and ultimately the world. The policy emphasized how the project would instill "new feelings of respect" in girls. Additionally, girls would develop a "love of sports," as well as new positive feelings about their bodies. Classes focused especially on helping girls find "pleasure" in their bodies through healthy exercise and movement, termed *harakat al-gism* (movements of the body) by the policy. The new hygienic practices, *nadafa*, included showers after sports activities. Policy described this as essential, because removing dirt and sweat from the body was critical to youth remaining healthy. Other practices were heralded as critical to the formation of healthy youth. Eating breakfast before playing sports was deemed essential to maximizing bodily health, and aid recipients also received training in appropriate dress (*libs*). They were encouraged to wear loose-fitting pants outside of the home, instead of the long robes they currently donned, so that they could have unrestricted movement of their legs during sports and games. Long skirts, the typical village dress for girls, were described as preventing girls' healthy movement.

These new practices of *harakat al-gism, nadafa,* and *libs* were described in policy as advancing "the right to play." The policy asserted that once girls understood and nurtured this right, which entailed the adoption of the new healthy habits described above, they would have a new relationship with their bodies and a new sense of self. They would ostensibly enjoy their bodies more, feel pleasure through them, and attain a new sense of youth selfhood.

Space figured centrally in this policy. Girls' bodily enjoyment was structured along a spatialized distinction between the indoors—described as oppressive—versus the outdoors, or the public realm—where emancipation and freedom were located. This spatial distinction was overwhelmingly gendered. It was asserted in the policy that boys already possessed the right to play and to enjoy freedom of movement in the public realm. The project sought to intervene on this convention and bring this right to girls as well. The literature, media, and pamphlets that circulated between aid offices about the project heavily promoted this spatial aspect of the project. Reports featured groundbreaking statistics about village girls occupying public youth centers for the very first time in Egyptian history, with images depicting village girls kicking soccer balls in sunny outdoor settings. This discourse was accompanied by testimonies from girls and aid workers about the project's successful outcomes. In the images, veiled girls wore loose pants, kicked soccer balls to each other, and had smiles on their faces. One media pamphlet emphasized the moral dimension of this fun, describing precisely how "girls enjoyed kicking the ball to one another and relished the vigorous exercise."

On the other side of the moral dimension were feelings of shame, which were associated in the policy and media with domestic confinement. Shame, the policy warned, was an unhealthy aspect of adolescence. Youthful sports activities conducted outdoors, described as natural and playful, and a source of liberation and girl empowerment, were the remedy for this shame. Similarly, statements from one policy report elaborated on how *harakat al-gism* could combat shame and instill new sensibilities in girls: "Activities such as jumping jacks, running, and kicking soccer balls helped girls feel more comfortable with their bodies—of particular importance during puberty when many girls, having been subjected to physical confinement, may not feel comfortable enjoying their bodies and finding expression through them. The sports component was designed to build girls' confidence and sense of ownership of their bodies."

Another media publication reiterated the importance of outdoor sports to shaping healthy selfhood for girls, positioning girls and boys against each other with respect to experiences of domestic confinement and occupying public space: "Rural girls work long hours in the home. […] Fears for their social reputation restrict mobility and community participation. Girls have little access to or time for recreation. Only five percent of rural girls reported having played sports in the previous day compared to fifty-six percent of boys."

As this excerpt makes clear, IVGP discourse asserted that traditional norms were obstacles to girls' recreational practices, their "right to play" sports. This same report asserted that for girls, religious fundamentalism was an underlying problem, inasmuch as it infringed on girls' healthy mobility. It suggested that intervention in these traditional norms by the IVGP would have a progressive and positive "ripple effect" in villages. Once villagers got accustomed to seeing girls in public, this visibility would become normalized, causing a general loosening of gender restrictions. This logic connected individual girls' bodies to village populations, and stipulated that the re-placement of girls' bodies could reshape village norms. Like the famous humanitarian slogan "Educate a girl, save a country," this aid discourse positioned village girls as panaceas for entire communities and nations. In the IVGP they were constructed as an antidote to village moral and cultural underdevelopment.

In sum, IVGP policy promoted village girl emancipation through the inculcation of new rights-driven practices that would then serve as remedies for girls' domestic confinement and exposure to "harmful traditions." Moving girls' bodies out of the home and into the public realm was key. Mobility, in the project, signaled, for girls, a move towards empowerment and entry into normative, global youthfulness. Yet it also signaled forward movement for entire villages, reflecting development discourse's emphasis on progression towards modernity. The "right to play" was a related tenet of the project. It separated girls from women, and was framed as essential to the relinquishing of feelings of shame for girls and to their experiencing pleasure in their own bodies. Villages, in the IVGP discourse, were depicted as marginalized spaces, places of rural otherness that were reeling from harmful religious conservatism and traditional values, whose greatest victims were adolescent girls. The aid professionals and administrators I spoke with and observed in Cairo while researching the IVGP held many of these views about Egyptian villages. Yet their personal and professional attachments to the project differed in significant ways, to which I now turn.

THE POLITICS OF IVGP AID WORKERS

This section highlights the perspectives and desires of the local aid workers who implemented the IVGP in Egypt. My conversations with these workers revealed a range of sentiments about the project. Workers had nuanced and competing ideas about what their work was doing for the girls, their communities, and Egypt as a nation. In the florescent-lit offices of the USDI, situated on the top floor of a tall business complex in downtown Cairo, I settled into a daily routine of assisting USDI administrators, demographers, and other office staff with their daily bureaucratic tasks. My job was to distribute memos, proofread reports, and organize stacks of paperwork that would eventually be distributed to staff prior to department meetings or field site visits. In addition, I assisted with refreshments during office meetings, or ran errands at nearby supermarkets that would help alleviate work for the receptionists or administrative assistants. As I completed these tasks, I interviewed and observed office staff as they went about their day-to-day activities. Grateful for the hospitality this staff showed me every day, I tried to make myself as useful as possible. They answered my questions and tolerated me as an ever-present, and overly eager, intern. The office resembled that of any typical corporate space. It constituted an entire floor of the building and had sectioned off spaces dedicated to various departments, including a corner relegated solely for child and youth humanitarian initiatives in Egypt.

Departments were relatively self-sufficient, and the office's director, an Egyptian-born social scientist with a doctoral degree, frequently traveled to the organization's headquarters in the United States or to Europe for meetings on global aid. For me, the office work was steady and relatively undemanding, freeing me up to chat with workers during extended office breaks, or to sit across from their desks discussing their roles in the IVGP. Workers were a close-knit group of young experts and professionals, predominantly Egyptian or of Arab heritage, who were passionate about their work advancing global aid initiatives like the IVGP. The majority of these workers were proficient in Arabic, English, and French, held a master's or doctoral degree, and were trained in fields relatively similar to my own, such as sociology, economics, international relations, or political science. Some were married and settled in Cairo, with young and growing families of their own, while others were attempting to spearhead transnational careers in international development or global health. The professional experiences they hoped to accrue while at USDI would, they believed, help them secure upper administrative jobs in the industry in one of many major European or American cities. As I worked in USDI, several large-scale initiatives were under way in the office, but soon after I arrived, I immediately spent the majority of my time working with the IVGP staff because theirs was among the most highly funded project. This group of five highly trained and motivated colleagues were responsible for producing knowledge about the project, making field site visits to villages, writing and securing grants, and overseeing local trainers who assisted village girls and ran the life-skills classes.

When it came to bringing the IVGP to Egyptian villages, which entailed recruiting girl participants and inaugurating the life-skills classes at local village youth centers, staff were quick to point out that they encountered friction on the ground, especially family resistance to the project. In addition, each worker had a different professional and personal background, which gave them different perspectives on village girls, as well as the experience of working on the project. In particular, they had conflicting views about the project's feasibility, its potential to produce its stated outcomes and successes, and what "care" meant with respect to village girls' health and welfare. Overall, the project meant something different to each aid worker, even as they all shared the fundamental belief that village girls were among the country's most vulnerable social group.

Aid workers focused their discussions about the project around two main themes. The first was the project's slow implementation in villages. In general, it was difficult for workers to get classes started and secure participants. The other theme that emerged in my discussions was the ethical attachment workers had to village girls, including sentiments about gender relations and the project's broader moral imperatives. The theme of national progress and development frequently arose with respect to the project's overall effects.

Regarding the first theme, workers faced what they saw as incredible hurdles from families when they attempted to recruit girls. Families outright resisted the project, and all the aid workers discussed how difficult a problem this was. They had to "work hard" to cultivate long-term relationships of trust and familiarity with family elders before they were willing to give girls permission to join the classes. Yasmine was one aid worker who helped secure girl participants in Beni Suef. She personally experienced the challenge of family resistance to the project. I asked her where the resistance to the project came from and how she managed it. "It was very difficult for families," she stressed, "because the project would expose girls to unrelated boys and men for the first time in their lives." In reflecting further upon this roadblock, she discussed how her recruitment efforts and unfailing commitment to "help" the girls eventually proved successful, but not without tiring persistence:

We encountered a lot of resistance at first, from the families, especially fathers. We knew we had to be persistent and keep showing up, reassuring them that the girls would be supervised, that they would not be in the presence of boys or men, that this project would have great benefits for the girls and the entire family. But you know, in the villages, it is difficult to change their ways, to convince them of things. They are very very strict. Our plan was to just keep pushing and pushing for these girls.

Yusef, another IVGP aid worker, shared a similar view. But when we spoke his responses indicated that for him, villages were radically different from major cities like Cairo, where he grew up, lives, and works. When I asked him how he dealt with recruitment problems and the fact that families resisted the project, he spoke about the inherent gaps in education in villages, the underdevelopment they suffer, and the "ideas" that plague people there. In addition to recruiting girl participants, his job, as he saw it, was also to educate villagers about their rural predicaments. "People there, they don't know they have problems," he explained. "We must go and enter their homes and explain to them what their problems are."

Yusef described how he dealt with resistance. He was able to successfully recruit girls through persistent negotiations with powerful family elders. By simply being "persistent" and present in the villages over long periods of time, he was able eventually to sway parents into allowing girls access to the classes. The reason families resisted the IVGP project so intensely was exposure, he claimed. Girls, they feared, would be exposed to unrelated boys and adult men in public, which would then put them in danger, or compromise their reputations in a society that placed high value on modest female behavior. Yusef described how in order to address this problem of exposure, project directors arranged for the banning of boys and men in local youth centers while IVGP classes were in session. This, he asserted, granted village girls a degree of privilege over public space that they had previously lacked. Aid workers labeled the time in which girls had sole access to youth centers as a "safe space" for women and girls only. By emphasizing to families how youth centers constituted "safe spaces" for girls, Yusef was able to recruit new participants and mitigate a major obstacle to the project's ongoing success. Lauding classes as gendered "safe spaces" meant girls were able to retain a level of privacy outside of the domestic realm. But, as Yusef went on to explain, convincing families in villages to take that risk still took time and effort, and repeated attempts at convincing elders that boys and men would not be present: "It was important that we made the parents know there would be no young men in the youth center during classes when the girls would be there. But this took a great deal of effort on our part. We had to earn their trust."

Yusef's comments and efforts to recruit girl participants for the IVGP illustrated how he saw himself as different from the villagers he worked with, as possessing a set of privileged and progressive ideas related to rights and gender equity. Similarly, many other aid workers at USDI believed they had expert knowledge about global human rights that aid recipients lacked, particularly in villages. They saw themselves as educators of village communities, speaking and acting on behalf of girls in the name of universal rights.

Along with the difficulties they faced in recruiting girl participants, aid workers had strong ethical attachments to the IVGP, and these attachments spoke to their special status as situated global aid experts. These attachments however were not identical. They varied according to each aid worker's subjectivity as well as their professional location within the organization. Accounts from Philippe, mentioned at the start of this chapter, Nadine, and Ihab, all IVGP aid workers, highlight some of these ethical disparities.

Philippe recalled how, growing up in Paris, he was always active in fighting for social justice and activism on behalf of Muslim immigrants. His intimate experiences with French immigration politics and the plight of marginalized Muslims in France fostered a long-standing personal interest in the Middle East and North Africa. After graduating in Paris with a political science degree, he delved into the world of international aid, first by volunteering at various nonprofits in Paris and eventually by securing paid positions at prominent global aid organizations. As a paid global aid worker, he immediately began working on Middle East and North Africa initiatives in the region, which frequently targeted vulnerable children and youth. He had lived in Egypt for several years while working for one such initiative. That immersive experience helped him develop crucial Arabic language skills and the local field knowledge necessary to join the IVGP staff at USDI's Cairo office once the project was in its inaugural phase.

During an interview, Philippe expressed fond memories of his time living in Cairo while working for the IVGP. When he had the chance to visit field sites in villages, whether to gather personal accounts of the project's success from recipients or produce statistics about village life, he felt connected to the girl recipients. These on-the-ground fieldwork experiences and observations gave Philippe special insights into village life that were not represented in formal global aid policy. They instilled in Philippe a critical perspective on how recipients were represented in the discourse of Western-based aid organizations. Spending time in villages, Philippe observed aid recipients behave as active subjects, as resilient and "strong" when faced with insurmountable structural inequality. He watched children and youth negotiate daily life and maximize opportunities so that they could improve their living conditions. But in the aid discourse, he asserted, these same youngsters are stripped of their abilities to act on their own behalf and are depicted as powerless, "the most vulnerable people in society. Even more vulnerable than women."

Philippe was particularly concerned about the deployment of racial and cultural stereotypes in global aid policy. He confessed that when it came to projects in Africa and the Middle East, global aid organizations relied heavily on Western fears of Islam, or what he termed Islamophobia, for funding purposes. During his time working in Egypt, he observed "the oppressed Muslim girl" serving as a resounding call for humanitarian action from people around the world. In his words, the figure of the Muslim girl helped a larger "fight against Islamic extremism." Having worked in the grant-writing departments of aid organizations, he had witnessed how organizations effectively communicated this call through images of vulnerable Muslim girls. Images such as a veiled child conveyed religious conservatism and traditionalism in its most glaring form. "It's the evidence of suffering that matters," he stressed when explaining these images. He went on to speak more about the power of gendered humanitarian images: "Come on, who could see those images and deny the aid or the help? You know that saying 'When the ship is sinking, children and women first.' Children are the future, [and] whenever the present is at risk, whenever there is a crisis, the first thing is the need to protect and preserve our future."

Here, Philippe referenced the notion, common in global aid representational regimes, that children are the future. Since they embody futurity, they are good "investments," Liisa Malkki has argued. Children deployed in this manner represent national hope, but they are also paradoxically depoliticized and universalized as pure sufferers and victims, as infantilized subjects, "relegated to the realm of the mere."[20]

Philippe's voice carried a tinge of sarcasm as he uttered the words, "children are the future." He was uncomfortable with the idea that children should be marked off as responsible for the future and that adults needed to save them in order to craft their ideal future utopia. His critique illustrated a clash between professional and personal obligations; they seemed strikingly at odds with each other. I asked Philippe how he negotiated the discord between his responsibilities at work and his personal views about humanitarian representations of young recipients. Philippe pointed to the monetary value racialized representations have in aid policy. He had this to say about the larger global economic "system" in which this affective work takes place:

> The poor African or Muslim girl brings aid money like no one else. Yes we use this to our advantage but it's the only way we can get funding. We have to use a stereotype to get money. This "clash of civilizations" story, Islam versus Christianity, using pictures of veiled Muslim girls. [...] I hate that stuff, but it brings [in] the money. I know it's exploitation, I know exactly what it is, but we have to play the politics. The funds keep the work going, we have to reach out and get them [funds] any way we can. We have to work with these politics and this system.

As this powerful statement makes clear, Philippe fiercely contested the use of racialized images that promoted aid projects and secured funding for organizations. Often in our conversations, he would refer to France's legacy as a colonial power in the Middle East and Africa, drawing on the unequal global relationship that continues to shape contemporary politics and aid relations between world regions. Philippe situated himself, as a Frenchman working in global aid, within these global predicaments and expressed great unease at what he thought was his complicit position. His narrative sheds light on how aid workers routinely grapple with reconciling their professional obligations with their personal politics.

Philippe's perspective also reveals tensions within large global aid processes that link international donors with individual aid workers who have intimate contact with recipients and who witness realities that are far more complex than the aid policy would communicate. His fierce criticism of the use of racialized images and his reluctance to approach village girls exclusively through their victim status in order to generate funding point to his ambivalent role in an aid system that relies on governments and corporate funders. As an outspoken advocate for social justice, Philippe did not hesitate to express his moral opposition to the same aid system in which he was complicit and on which he was dependent for his own professional advancement.

Philippe's views can be juxtaposed with those of Nadine, an IVGP project manager who had overwhelmingly positive responses to my questions about the initiative and whose personal obligations were very much aligned with those of the project. Of all the aid workers I spoke with, she was the IVGP's biggest supporter. Nadine celebrated any global aid initiative that focused on village girls in Africa and the Middle East. She helped write the policy for the IVGP and believed the initiative was not only a necessary intervention, but it was an unprecedented, benevolent move on the part of global aid organizations, which had previously focused on either women's or children's welfare. Leaning back in her office chair one day, she talked about the IVGP's many groundbreaking successes, "These girls are now enlightened, they have life skills!" She continued to describe the positive transformation village girls in Egypt experienced as a result of their participation in the project, "Before, these girls would have never been able to travel or leave the area where they lived. Now, they can go to school and that is a major achievement!" This was a critical shift for Nadine. Witnessing girls move from domestic to public life gave her a deep sense of personal accomplishment, and not only professional achievement.

The sentimental attachments and affinity Nadine had for village girls was, according to her, rooted in her personal background. She was of Algerian heritage, and had been working at USDI Cairo on other gender-based initiatives for over a decade before I joined the office. She had a master's degree in sociology from a French university and a long history of social activism throughout her education. While she was working on her graduate degree, she did a year of fieldwork on child labor in Egypt. That formative experience facilitated her first exposure to children's experiences with extreme poverty in Cairo and gave her important insights into how children navigated economic and labor exploitation. During this fieldwork, she collaborated with a network of global aid organizations in Cairo, allowing her to forge lasting professional relationships with USDI aid workers. Upon graduating with her master's degree, she landed an administrative job at USDI in Cairo and, over the years, worked her way up within the organization to occupy a very coveted and respected institutional position, that of project director.

Nadine was fluent in Arabic, French, and English. Multilingualism, she reminded me, was highly valued by global aid upper administrators, because knowledge flowed transnationally to and from aid offices in the global north and south. Professionally, as a trilingual aid expert, Nadine acted as a critical intermediary between USDI offices in France, Africa, the United States, and the Middle East. Personally, Nadine considered herself to be both Arab and francophone, viewing herself as having to negotiate a dual subjectivity at work with her Egyptian colleagues. When it came to her professional life in Cairo, she believed she was both an insider and an outsider, not quite foreign, as Arab, but also not quite local. This ambiguous status sometimes made social life difficult for her in Cairo, but she believed it served her exceptionally well professionally and situated her as an expert who was culturally malleable and, as she explained it, "not rooted" in one particular place, as someone who had a bird's-eye view when it came to Egypt. As she put it, her foreign Arab identity made it possible for her to "see the country's social problems that maybe an Egyptian wouldn't be able see."

In the office, Nadine was a well-respected authority figure. Other aid workers deferred to her as the "person in charge" of the IVGP. As its first project manager, she helped launch the IVGP across southern Egypt, inaugurating the first set of classes herself. During the time I worked in the office, I watched Nadine secure a follow-up grant for the IVGP and make multiple trips to villages where she oversaw classes, interviewed girls, and ensured that local trainers were following formal aid policy procedures. These trips allowed her to maintain enduring relationships with girl participants. Upon arriving back in Cairo from one such village trip, Nadine spoke to me about the girls she had just interviewed, emphasizing the profound effect the classes were having on their lives and the ways in which the girls "changed" after participating in the project. Nadine also spoke about the changes she was experiencing herself as an aid worker responsible for transforming girls' lives and enacting this lasting change: "I believe in this project. And I am so proud of those girls. When you first see them, they can't even leave their home or village. They are so shy. Then they change, they gain these life skills and they learn about their bodies, they talk about things they couldn't speak about before and they become somebody. You see them more independent, more open, more enlightened. You then feel good about yourself."

For Nadine, the IVGP was emancipatory not only for girl recipients but for aid workers like herself as well. In contrast to Philippe's critique of global aid politics and the humanitarian uses of racialized images of Muslim girls in order to secure grants, Nadine's sentiments lauded global aid efforts to uplift and empower village girls. She firmly believed they were agentless victims, and that the project was performing important, ethical work in villages where girls were underserved in terms of resources, compassion, and rights. She saw herself and other USDI workers as offering this critical, necessary care.

Nadine's ideas about the IVGP reinforced the notion that village girls were pure sufferers who were exposed to gender violence and religious conservatism in their communities. These ideas reflected the global policy discourses she herself helped create. She considered herself an advocate for disempowered women and girls across the Middle East and harbored a strong professional impulse to act on their behalf. With her personal roots in the region, she saw herself as a francophone Arab feminist. To this end, she believed the project was advancing girls' empowerment, even if in a limited and incremental manner. From breaking out of their shyness to leaving the physical confines of their homes, village girls, Nadine passionately pointed out to me in our conversations, were powerfully changed forever by IVGP interventions. Having benefited from a Western education and lived what she termed "feminist ideals" throughout her life, Nadine was optimistic about what the IVGP could do for girl aid recipients. The self-esteem girls seemed to convey to her when she visited them to discuss the project was palpable, she emphasized. She believed that, as a result of the classes and rights-based interventions the project was bringing to villages, girls could finally "make something out of themselves and improve their own lives."

Ihab, a Cairo native from an upper-middle-class, rather cosmopolitan family in his early forties, represents another thread in a web of relationships engendered by the IVGP between aid workers, families, and village girls. As a demographer, his job responsibilities at USDI included managing financials and monitoring budgets associated with the IVGP. Ihab had an extensive personal and professional travel history. He had vacationed, lived, and worked in Europe and the United States and earned a college degree in London before settling into a career in global development aid in Cairo. This global experience and transnational outlook, nurtured by a top-notch education in London, informed his desire to "develop" Egypt in the image of Western countries. One afternoon, early in my research, we spoke about the IVGP's aims in Egypt. Ihab identified the source of village girl suffering as the "village" context itself, and believed that villages were rife with problems that held Egypt back in the world. Villages, he believed, contributed to Egypt's global status as an "undeveloped" country, they were a source of the nation's economic and political problems.

When we spoke about the IVGP, Ihab often juxtaposed the urban with the rural, describing the latter through othering discourses of Islamic extremism and religious repression. In English, he would often talk about the village as being "over there" and the city as being "here," the place where "we are." One day, when I was in the office preparing for my first trip to Beni Suef to meet IVGP girl aid recipients, Ihab reminded me that I needed to cover my hair upon arrival, especially if I were in the presence of men. "But since you're a foreigner," he fervently stated, pointing to his forehead, "you can show a little hair in front, but be sure to cover up the rest!" This caveat about my modest presentation in the village spoke to Ihab's concern for my welfare and safety "in the field," as most USDI aid workers referred to villages. But it also reiterated his belief that things were radically different "over there" in villages, so much so that I needed to take precautions there that were presumably unnecessary in Cairo. Although veiling is not required of women in Egyptian villages, Ihab's caveat conveyed the sense that it was the norm, and therefore somewhat expected of me.

Ihab's discourse linking villages to national development was rather common among aid workers at USDI, reflecting ideas about rural otherness that Timothy Mitchell, in writing about rural Egypt and urban representations of peasant subjectivity, were constructed by experts for urban consumption. Such representations of the village remain devoid of colonial histories or contemporary state policies that produced and sustain the idea of underdevelopment. Moreover, these representations, as they continue to circulate in the world of global development aid, operate under the assumption that "villagers" are the timeless objects of development and urban middle classes are separate from them, or ostensibly more "civilized."[21]

Ihab believed that village development was essential if Egypt was to achieve national progress, and that village girls were, at present, the means through which this steady, incremental process of movement would occur, if ever. Surprisingly, however, Ihab believed that village girls were not the most vulnerable population in Egypt. He elaborated, "If you go to the villages, you'll see, these are actually happy girls." Other workers who made field visits to villages also referred to girl recipients as "relaxed" and "smiling." For Ihab then, Islamic fundamentalism, conservatism, and poverty were more urgent problems than the suffering of one social group, girls, because those greater structural forces held villages "back," and therefore kept Egypt from progressing in the image of Western Europe or the United States.

While IVGP policy framed village girls as innocent victims and harbingers of a better, more enlightened future, Ihab believed it would be larger national and economic transformations that would push the country forward. He referenced the need for infrastructure in villages and more investment in education. But, in echoing Philippe's previous critique of global aid, Ihab stressed that structural causes did not generate significant donor funds for organizations like the USDI. Rather, it was the appeal to urgent suffering, such as the plight of adolescent village girls, that propelled international support. Ihab believed that eventually, however, the resources from the IVGP would "trickle down" from girls to their larger communities, and that this ripple effect would precipitate broader structural changes in villages. For Ihab, therefore, something was better than nothing when it came to the procurement of resources, and, in this sense, girls, as a humanitarian category, were a salient social group for the organization and a means to achieve national development goals.

In reflecting upon Ihab's perspectives, I came to understand that the IVGP was a burgeoning humanitarian intervention focused on village girls as well as a strategy of national development, one that would ostensibly carry Egypt towards the goal of national progress. For him, it was a significant project because it could help raise Egypt's human rights and development index on par with that of Western countries. In addition, it could help propel the country's cultural advancement, even if it was through the education and uplifting of a singular population—out-of-school adolescent village girls. For Ihab, cultural advancement, whether through education or the inculcation of human rights, was instrumental to reinforcing a cosmopolitan, middle-class subjectivity in Egypt. It was a subjectivity that stood in stark contrast with that of the villager. As Partha Chatterjee notes in the case of postcolonial India, development initiatives in postcolonial contexts have helped to promote and reproduce a dominant national identity that is essentially urban and middle-class, and the IVGP was viewed by Ihab as instrumental to this process taking hold in Egyptian villages.[22]

THE EXPERIENCE OF VILLAGE GIRLS: HIBA AND SHAYMA

An approximately three-hour drive south from Cairo leads to miles of verdant agricultural land punctuated by majestic palm trees, the Nile River, and eventually, the southern Egyptian governorate of Beni Suef. Lying on the border between Lower and Upper Egypt, the region is described in state and development discourse as having some of the highest levels of poverty in the country, along with some of the fastest growth in the number of out-of-school girls. Water and sanitation remain major concerns in the region, along with unemployment and basic social services such as healthcare and public education. While accompanying me into Beni Suef, Ali, a local USDI worker who helped facilitate projects in the area, described the dearth of job opportunities for young men as a result of neglect on the part of the state, with "no big business projects happening here." In my interviews with Ali and families in Beni Suef, poverty and the lack of jobs available for young people emerged time and again as dominant themes. Yet a heavy and steady influx of foreign and local aid into the region continues, defining the governorate as a development crisis zone. The official number of state-registered NGOs in Beni Suef in 2010 was four thousand, a figure that has likely increased since then. As a favored site for experiments like the IVGP because of its exceptional status as a development crisis zone, Beni Suef was steeped in aid interventions in 2008. However, a rise in NGO development interventions did not secure better livelihoods for locals. Due to a steady increase in poverty, everyday life for villagers has not improved, and statistics depict a rise in unemployment and the number of out-of-school children. During the day, most out-of-school girls perform domestic labor or work in the fields tending crops, while their brothers attend public schools, which in Egypt still require that families pay a range of informal fees. Owing to the rising cost of living, many households struggle to meet these fees.

Upon arriving at the local youth center, I immediately met with Hiba, who was twelve years old. She already graduated from an earlier installment of the IVGP and was now assisting current participants with classes. Reminiscing about her time in class, she spoke nostalgically about how important she felt when she and the other girls in class "took over" the youth center. As she recalled, "We never get that. We had the space all to ourselves. We came first, before the boys. We felt special and we liked it very much." While she spoke, we sat in a room in the youth center where her classes took place. The center itself was a run-down, empty shell of a building that at the time of its construction in the 1970s served a more central role in the community. Now, it was mostly a communal meeting point where entire families gathered for public prayers or to celebrate Ramadan. Colorful murals adorned its concrete walls on the outside depicting young men and women performing physical activities and youthful exercises: they lifted weights, swam, and kicked soccer balls. Inside, the building was spacious, cold, and empty. The sounds of our voices echoed off of the brightly painted walls, and meandering corridors eventually led us to a main hall where large events took place.

Back in the classroom where we talked, Hiba shifted in her chair and told us what she had learned from the IVGP project. She emphasized the new habits she had developed through the classes, such as how she had to eat breakfast on the days when she had sports training, and how she took a shower afterwards in order to become "clean" (*nadifa*). Echoing the formal policy aims, she mentioned how important it was for her to stop wearing long robes and instead wear loose-fitting floor-length pants so that she could play sports and move around freely. Hiba also mentioned how much she enjoyed gathering with her classmates for the classes, and how "free" the project made her feel. She beamed as she thoughtfully described the classes, and the enthusiasm was written all over her face. The newly inculcated habits she talked about seemed to reflect the project's stated successes precisely as they appeared in IVGP policy.

Later that day, Hiba and I met with a small group of five current IVGP participants. A tight-knit group of friends, they ranged in age from twelve to sixteen years old. Although they were new students, they shared Hiba's enthusiasm for the project and commented on the fun, social aspects of the classes. We sat in a circle in the youth center classroom, sipping fruit juice boxes and discussing their time in class as well as my background—a subject of much curiosity. "Are you married?" Shayma', the most outspoken girl in the group, probed. I tried to ignore the look of confusion on each girl's face after I responded that no, I was not and never had been. I was visibly much older than the girls, a fact that made my unmarried status odd, even abnormal, because marriage marks proper entry into moral adulthood in Egypt. Feeling uncomfortable with the attention, I attempted to change the subject by asking questions about the IVGP classes, but marriage, I soon realized, was what this group was interested in discussing.

Early marriage and domestic labor were labeled two global human rights "abuses" that the IVGP targeted for eradiation. Yet these were aspects of village social life that remained unaltered by the IVGP. Ironically, the girls I spoke with in Beni Suef placed a particularly high value on marriage. They saw themselves as agents in the process of finding a marriage partner or active decision-makers in the process of declining a marriage prospect. A few hours later, Hiba's older sister joined us for a bit. She brought her baby—a bubbly, cheerful infant girl wrapped in layers of plush blanket—but soon left her with us in order to tend to other business. As we continued to chat, I noticed Hiba passing the baby around the circle to the other girls. It seemed her arms and shoulders had gotten tired. Each girl picked up the baby for a few minutes before passing her on to the next nearby friend. Soon, my interview questions about the IVGP became overshadowed by the giddy sounds of the infant and the excitement generated by her presence. The girls knew this baby well and appeared eager to contribute to her care. Soon, perhaps bored, they shifted the conversation away from the IVGP classes and onto the baby. Eventually, we began talking about marriage and courtship in the village. Rather than stick to my prepared, structured interview questions, I was delighted to let the girls shape the contours of our conversation as they wished.

In facilitating my entry into the village, Ali had mentioned that marriage was a topic that was, "always on the minds of the youth," in Beni Suef. Remembering his words, I noticed the girls light up at the talk of marriage in the village. They exchanged comments about who was getting married to whom, when and how the families would find the money for the wedding. Three of the six girls in the group that afternoon had already been engaged at some point in their lives. They spoke about these previous engagements as a source of value and pride, as a reflection of their status as desirable subjects. Together, as a group, they expressed anxieties over the possibility of their marriages being delayed. Hiba recalled how one young couple that year had to tragically call off their wedding because the families could not afford the high cost of the wedding.

Sometimes, however, delayed marriages in the village occurred less because of economic constraints and more because of a lack of chemistry between young couples. Shayma' was sixteen and had previously been engaged. She shared how she had decided to break off her engagement to a suitor who was three years her senior because he wasn't acting jealous enough around her. For her, *ghir* (jealousy) was an expression of a man's attraction to and interest in his beloved. Her fiancé's apparent lack of jealously rendered him less attractive to her as marriage partner. When I shared with Shayma' that jealously was commonly perceived as a negative trait where I came from, she said, "If a man doesn't express jealously for a girl, it's obvious he doesn't like her enough. That's why I broke it [wedding] off with my fiancé." Shayma' explained that she now had a new fiancé. I asked if this new young man was a more suitable partner, and she responded with a resounding, "Yes, he's jealous!" and invited me to her upcoming wedding, the date to which had not been determined.

As Shayma''s views about marriage illustrate, rather than expressing an aversion to marriage, girls in Beni Suef seemed to look forward to their wedding days and believed they had a considerable amount of agency in the process. They even communicated deep-seated fears as well as a level of anxiety over the possibility that their weddings would be delayed due to economic constraints. Shayma''s relationship to her suitors and overall perspectives on marriage contrasted sharply with IVGP discourse. Aid policy described aid recipients like Shayma'' as helpless victims and marriage as a child-rights violation. According to the girls, the project succeeded in providing them with mobility beyond domestic spaces and it instilled new feelings of freedom into them. However, our unexpected conversation in the youth center revealed that it seemed to have little to no effect on their views of marriage.

In addition to views about marriage, domestic labor—a practice that was targeted for eradication by the IVGP—persisted in girls' lives after their participation in the IVGP. Previously established routines, which included household chores, continued for the girls while classes were in session as well. In other words, kinship and household obligations were not eradicated, but coexisted with the new arrangements and relationships engendered by the project. For instance, as she was participating in the project, Shayma' described how she had to wake up much earlier than usual in order to complete her household chores before making it to class on time at the local youth center. Although she admitted that this was physically taxing for her, she willingly complied because she enjoyed the classes; they kept her active and involved with other participants. They offered her a break from her usual routine, an opportunity to make new girlfriends, and, as she stressed, they created in her new feelings of "freedom" (*hurriya*). She went on to explain her new routine: "I had to wake up at 5:00 or 5:30 in the morning instead of later on. I had to finish all my house chores before I could leave for the lessons at 9:00 a.m. Yes, I was tired but I liked it. I felt free and like no one could rule over me." For Shayma', the mobility and feelings of independence she gained from the project did not supplant her obligations in her household. Rather, they overlapped with them, adding to her workload. Though the classes made her life more difficult in a practical sense, Shayma' welcomed the added stress because she gained other benefits from the project and "liked it."[23]

Hiba and Shayma''s experiences were just two among many in Beni Suef that demonstrated how the IVGP had unanticipated and paradoxical effects for girls. I do not wish to imply that the project was outright harmful for these girls, but nor do I suggest that it was wholly benevolent, at least in the ways that it purported itself to be. What I am implying instead is a more subtle approach to how, in practice, the IVGP produced effects that did not fit into either of these categories. For instance, it did not address, in any aspect of its intervention, the social and economic conditions structuring domestic labor for girls in villages, or why marriage aspirations among girls are so persistent and central to what it means to be an adolescent girl. As IVGP participants, Hiba and Shayma' enjoyed certain aspects of the project, including the new avenues of sociality and mobility opened up by the classes. Each girl reconciled her newly established responsibilities and sense of "freedom" with her existing household obligations and personal sentiments. The new knowledge and sensibilities they gained did not produce adverse effects other than more work or physical exhaustion. Hiba and Shayma' reiterated to me how "special" and "free" they felt because of the classes.

When we last spoke, Shayma' shared how excited she was about her new fiancé, contradicting one of the project's ultimate goals—the eradication of early marriage. Her desire to be married and her affectionate feelings for her new fiancé unsettled many of the dominant humanitarian representations of Muslim village girls as helpless victims of early marriage and traditional practices. Whether or not this was the case, Hiba and Shayma' seemed less concerned about marrying too young than about the poverty in their village and the ways in which economic insecurity affected their families' ability to pay for their weddings. They did not perceive their vulnerabilities as girls as separate from or greater than those of their families, brothers, or communities. Eager to leave their homes and develop new skills, they neither rejected nor wholly embraced the practices and habits conveyed to them through IVGP classes. Nonetheless, aid policy defined them in terms of pure innocence and agentless suffering,[24] which had powerful effects on USDI's grant funding and project expansion, notwithstanding that it did not reflect Hiba and Shayma''s more complicated lived experience.

CONCLUDING THOUGHTS

The difficult question I have continued to grapple with after conducting research on the IVGP and after meeting girls like Hiba and Shyma unfortunately remains unanswered. How do we account for the discord between global aid efforts that focus exclusively on the health and welfare of village girls, in the Middle East and elsewhere, and which approach them as an exceptionally vulnerable humanitarian category, and the enduring collective suffering and structural violence in villages, suffering that requires complex, revolutionary, and protracted political and economic policy transformation? Must we choose between assisting girls and privileging community welfare in large-scale global aid projects? And where do we locate the nuanced perspectives of situated aid workers who are transnational experts that create and enact global aid policy, who perceive their work differently, and for whom village girls can constitute both pure victims but also agents who make decisions, are happy, and are not necessarily the most vulnerable group in their society? I began tracing the many people and discourses associated with the IVGP in Egypt in early 2007. Just as I was leaving the field in late 2009, I learned that the IVGP was undergoing a process of rapid expansion into other villages across Egypt, in Yemen, and sub-Saharan Africa. The transnational expansion of the project speaks to the powerful appeal village girls' suffering continues to have for donors, policy-makers, and aid experts in the industry.

This chapter has shed light on the grounded tensions and contradictions village girl projects produce in the context of Egypt—pointing to what global aid initiatives for village girls may actually do in other places as well. The Muslim village girl, that quintessential humanitarian object according to Philippe, was constructed in IVGP policy through the same timeless registers as the Muslim woman in development aid, yet she was given the added dimension of biological vulnerability, owing to puberty. In her society, the policy asserts, the liminal and dangerous biological state of puberty sets her apart from children and adult women, the other two primary global aid recipient groups, marking her as more vulnerable and in need of intervention. In IVGP discourse, girls were described as agentless innocent victims, as depoliticized, and as pure sufferers. They were given the universal status of "youth," yet they were also othered and described in terms of their rural, conservative Muslim identities. These representational, tranquilizing registers of vulnerability compelled urban audiences and donor institutions to act on village girls' behalf, to care about them, and to donate funds for their protection, uplift, and care. Rather than promote intervention into governmental policies, military systems, or the global markets that helped to sustain rural underdevelopment in Egyptian villages, global aid organizations like USDI deploy the Muslim village girl figure in aid policy as a distinct, worthy, and savable figure. This figure has helped organizations advance region-wide girl centered initiatives, and with much success.

Aside from speaking for Muslim village girls, and ascribing onto them a victim status which girls themselves challenge or complicate, there are other consequences that result from global aid initiatives of this kind. In a post–9/11 moment, when global fears about religious extremism abound, Muslim village girl aid initiative can deepen preexisting global anxieties about Islam and marginalized masculinities in the Middle East. In marking village girls as the worthiest objects of aid in Egypt because of their exposure to gender-based violence, organizations such as USDI implicitly mark local boys and men as the source of suffering. Thus, the saving of Muslim village girls in Egypt through the IVGP also entailed a moral and cultural disciplining, through global aid, of village boys, men, and community leaders. According to this logic, not only could village boys never constitute worthy objects of global aid in the same ways girls do, they are marked as suspicious or threatening subjects, and as a potential source of village girl oppression.

As the aid policy furthered these cultural and racial discourses about village communities, the professional and ethical orientations of IVGP aid workers revealed the diverse ways in which they approached the IVGP and villages in Egypt. As educated, multilingual experts whose identities did not neatly fall into an East/West binary, these aid workers were sometimes caught in a double bind, having to negotiate complex personal criticisms of the project with their work obligations, as was the case with Philippe, or with their national ambitions for development and progress, as Ihab illustrated. At other times, liberal feminist understandings of self-actualization and individual freedom drove their attachments to the project, as was the case with Nadine. Regardless of their underlying personal motives, professional obligations, or political subjectivities, aid workers in some way or other expressed a need to help, whether they believed it was village girls, villages, or the nation, that required their assistance.[25] They also experienced a process of self-transformation as a result of doing what they saw as generally good work through the IVGP. For workers like Ihab, self-transformation reinforced a middle-class, urban subjectivity that positioned him against a rural and religiously conservative other.[26] For self-proclaimed feminists like Nadine, assisting village girls produced good feelings within her, including a sense of pride in promoting gender empowerment among vulnerable girls in the region. In each instance, the outcomes of the grounded aid encounter were relational, a two-way process, rather than singular. This means that aid workers were shaped in some way through their aid work with village girls.[27]

In the following chapter, I carry these questions about how aid workers experience their work forward by focusing on the local experts who work for global aid organizations in Egypt and who craft national policy for vulnerable children.

Chapter 5

PROFESSIONAL AMBIVALENCE

SALMA HAD A PROFESSIONAL AND COMMANDING PRESENCE. SHE WAS tall, middle-aged, and dressed in a black pant suit and white head scarf when she entered the conference room one morning where I and a group of global aid workers had gathered. As a state minister, the degree of public formality with which she carried herself, both in attire and bodily comportment, was expected of her. She greeted us politely and then settled into the office chair that was positioned at the head of room. The aid workers sat directly in front of her in chairs that were thoughtfully organized in rows, like students facing their professor in class. We sat waiting for her first move. There was no question that Salma was in charge of this meeting. She seemed calm and in control, and all of our eyes were fixed on her. Then 'Adil, the organization's director, dutifully placed a cup of coffee in her hand. Salma sipped her coffee, and then, in a stern and confident tone, kicked off the meeting with a prepared speech. The focus was street children, and the message was clearly directed at the global aid workers seated before her:

> Who are we? And what is our work? And who are our children? We the government try to protect the individual child and the society because they are interconnected. We are here trying to help those addicted to drugs, because our kids haven't learned how to be strong and disciplined when faced with the decision of whether or not to take drugs. They have no tools at their disposal to help them resist, they haven't had anyone teach them. So, our

greatest and strongest relationship should be with parents. Our job is to teach these values. Our work is children, children without law. We have a responsibility to them.

Silence filled the room. Omar, the director of CCI's street children's shelter, who appears in chapter 3 of this book, was in attendance. He seemed fully engaged in what Salma said. With a firm, commanding voice, and sounding disturbed, he asked Salma a question related to the children's shelter that he oversees: "What is the government going to do about all the kids, the countless kids here with no parents, who live in a deplorable state? I have to take them in with the little I have. I need help!"

Salma immediately sat higher in her chair, appearing larger and more in charge of the meeting. She responded to Amir's question in a louder voice than his: "I have done my share and what I can, you must do yours. And you should refrain from thinking and speaking the way you do!"

Another extended moment of silence filled the room. Rana, an expert in humanitarian law, interjected in a lowered voice, in a show of deference. Her question to Salma sounded couched in desperation: "*Ustaza* [a title denoting respect towards a woman] if you permit, about the police who bring children to the centers in handcuffs as if they are adults, this is degrading and shameful. And harmful to children."

Rana lifted both of her hands up in the air for Salma to see. She clasped them at the wrists, mimicking the oppressive experience of being handcuffed. With her hands frozen in this position, she continued to address Salma: "It is unnecessary for policemen to handcuff a five-year-old boy like this and then throw him into the back of a vehicle with adults."

Other aid workers nodded their heads in agreement as they waited for Salma's response. Salma shifted again in her chair, and now sounded agitated: "Between us and the children there are a lot of problems! Officers have to do their job! They are not the ones who decide where the child goes. They simply bring the children to the detention center indiscriminately. Breaking the law and child protection are two different things! Plus, the children don't stay at the center very long, just up to a week or two. Then they are resituated in the proper institutions."

Upon hearing this, and like an avalanche, the aid workers collectively launched a string of complaints about the police. They were clearly dissatisfied with Salma's response and kept questioning the conditions inside detention centers. To them, Salma was the appropriate target for these complaints, because she was the figurehead, the face, of the state in front of them that day, and as a group they had harbored grievances about police mishandling of children for months, if not years. Their frustrations were now surfacing for all to see during this heated exchange.

As the complaints flew her way, Salma stubbornly defended her position with equal zeal, firing back at the workers with explanations about detention improvements and funding troubles. At one point in the exchange, Salma pointed a finger at the workers, as if to discipline them. The meeting seemed to spiral out of control, before Rana interrupted and announced, "Everyone, please, street children are Egypt's biggest problem. We should set aside our opinions and remember that!" The message quelled the exchange. Everyone, including Salma, nodded in agreement and refrained from further debate. Salma appeared as if she had reached her limit with the workers. She said her good-byes gracefully and then exited the conference room. The aid workers continued to discuss the difficulties children faced in detention centers even after Salma's departure. For several more minutes, they complained among themselves that state authorities keep evading their efforts to introduce reforms on behalf of street children.

This contentious encounter took place while I was interning in the Cairo branch of Global Aid for Children (GAC; the name has been changed to protect anonymity), a London-based organization that collaborated with CCI on humanitarian initiatives for street children in Egypt. Since the 1990s, GAC had been promoting healthcare as a human right for the child across the Middle East. As a prominent child-focused organization, it was also active around the world in promoting children's rights and in crafting national policies focused on child protection. Its Cairo branch was a major site in Egypt for child-focused medical aid and humanitarian work, which was why I interned there for much of 2008 and why key aid experts from various organizations were present to meet with Salma that morning.

Intimate encounters with high-ranking state employees like Salma were rare moments for these aid workers. As a network of professionals, they lacked opportunities to directly confront state actors together, and because they worked so closely with street children on a day-to-day basis, witnessing firsthand the effects of police violence against street children, they felt a great deal of accumulated pain and frustration. That pain and frustration surfaced in the meeting with Salma. If anything, it underscored a deeply interdependent and embattled relationship between the workers of global aid organizations and state actors. Workers scheduled the meeting in the first place because they had been advocating for new child-protection strategies (*himayat al-tifl*) for years following UNCRC guidelines. They encountered repeated roadblocks on this front, the biggest of which was ongoing police violence against street children. They hoped that by meeting with Salma, they could help sway a powerful administrator to finally promote new rights-based practices in places where street children were actually being detained and physically abused.

But the meeting tailed off into a dramatic reminder that global aid work in specific places produces what Anna Tsing called "frictions": the awkward, unequal, and unstable qualities of global interconnections.[1] Frictions are contingent, worldly encounters. They are messy and can lead to new arrangements of culture and power in particular sites. Similarly, enacting global aid policy on behalf of children in Egypt was messy, creative, and combative work for GAC aid experts. It often positioned them at the intersections of global and local knowledge claims and practices, and, as Salma's visit revealed, riddled their professional experiences with conflicts over child welfare. This was both compromising and empowering work for GAC professionals. It brought to light some of the key paradoxical dimensions of global medical aid for high-ranking experts situated at the level of international law and national policy-making. The ways in which aid workers interpreted power and authority in relation to Salma was indicative of how global aid organizations, in general, are figured precariously within state structures. Power shifts, overlaps, and co-exists in these relations. However, GAC aid workers always remained deferential to Salma and other state authorities in their attempts to promote new policies. Their deference pointed to the sense of ambivalence and vulnerability they shared while attempting to do the work of the state and that of global aid organizations.[2]

THE PARADOXICAL POSITION OF LOCAL AID EXPERTS

Who exactly are these aid administrators, lawyers, and child-rights experts who work in global aid offices on behalf of vulnerable children in Egypt? In this chapter, I focus on this question, and capture the narratives and practices of high-ranking aid experts. I approach them as critical actors in the story of global medical aid for children in Egypt. They are the professional "global citizens" who interpret international children's rights discourses and translate them into local policies and standardized practice.[3] Understanding their desires, challenges, and motivations sheds new light on the culture of global aid in Egypt and the politics of humanitarian policy-making for children.[4] In many ways, these workers resemble what Sally Engle Merry called the "cultural intermediaries" of globalization because they reconstitute international knowledge for local groups through a process of vernacularization.[5] For Merry, vernacularization requires that transnational elites like those at GAC reinterpret and reappropriate global discourses while reframing local stories into the global language of rights. This dual movement, as Merry has outlined for the case of human rights movements against gender violence, situates global aid workers at the interstices of the global/local imagined binary. However, this duality also creates invariable tensions for experts because they operate with a kind of "double consciousness" while they participate in two cultural spheres at once.

The concept of vernacularization resembles the daily work practices I witnessed at GAC. Aid experts attempted to understand and translate the tenets of children rights for national policies. As they did so, they were continually negotiating their professional identities and personal obligations at the intersections of state institutions, GAC's headquarters in London, and local groups who were fiercely critical of the cultural assumptions and moral claims inherent in international children's rights.

Salma's visit to GAC best exemplified how local realities can clash with the doctrines of international children's rights. This friction made the work of local aid experts like Rana taxing and even demoralizing. At times, Rana's professional goals seemed impossible for her to achieve. For her, vernacularization was a practice that was deeply fraught with ambivalences, contradictions, and inter-relational struggles over child welfare. Local authorities, including state ministers, the police, and even religious leaders, were her greatest obstacles to success in aid work. Their resistance to the new child-rights doctrines GAC was promoting prevented her from achieving what she believed were professional and personal outcomes at work.

After the meeting with Salma ended, I followed Rana out of the conference room into the employee lounge, where she usually prepared an afternoon cup of tea. She was clearly frustrated by the collective exchange with Selma, so I decided to check up on her. As I pulled a coffee mug out of the kitchen cabinet, Rana sprinkled some sugar into her teacup. "Do you think the meeting even accomplished anything?" I asked, hoping to hear some positive feedback. Rana replied with a sarcastic smile and a shake of her head, "Ha! I don't know. We'll just have to see."

Her demeanor indicated it had not. Rana went on to explain how she had spent months prior to Salma's visit translating Child Law amendments into Arabic for the ministry. On several occasions, she even made site visits to child detention facilities around Cairo, advocating for new legal amendments that would deter police brutality against children. One amendment sought to ban the imprisonment of children in adult prison cells. She was typically fully dedicated to child protection along these lines, and usually had an energetic and upbeat attitude in the office. But that morning, after Salma left, Rana expressed doubt that her contributions would even make a difference. Angst was written all over her face.

Rana's skepticism that day exemplified the kind of ambivalent relationship many GAC workers had towards their work with international children's rights. They believed in the promises of children's bodily integrity and justice as articulated in the doctrines of international children's rights, yet faced daily resistance in accomplishing the work, in seeing it actualized in real life. This resistance led them to doubt, and even criticize, the cultural underpinnings of children's rights and, more broadly, the end goals of global medical aid for children.

Despite these doubts, however, GAC workers remained fierce advocates for child welfare in Egypt, retaining high hopes for future political transformation through the vehicle of children's rights and the reforms they could engender while at GAC. For these reasons, they found themselves caught in what I saw as a professional paradox, one in which they actively promoted and undermined the underlying doctrines of international children's rights, viewing rights as both essential and inadequate for progress in the realm of child welfare.

THE RELATIONS BETWEEN GLOBAL AID ORGANIZATIONS AND THE STATE

As mentioned earlier, Salma's visit to GAC elucidated aspects of a broader state–global aid organization relationship in Egypt. GAC collaborated with governments across the global south to develop national policies focused on the bodies of "children at risk." In Egypt, these policies focusing on children first began to take hold in the 1990s, but GAC had roots in Egypt that spanned farther back. Since 1982, it had established offices in Egypt that sought to combine healthcare, education, and protection services together in order to advocate for vulnerable groups. In its policy for children, rights and bodily integrity were major themes. GAC purported to intervene in matters where children's physical and psychological well-being were threatened. It claimed that in 2008, Egypt had approximately thirty-five million vulnerable children who were at risk of these threats, an alarming figure. In GAC policy, child laborers, child refugees, and street children figured into the formal categorization of vulnerable children. The organization's funding came primarily from private-sector corporations such as ExxonMobil, Johnson & Johnson, and the Ford Foundation. However, various global political entities such as USAID, the United Nations, and the European Commission also provided substantial funding for its projects. In 2013, the organization estimated its total budget for Egypt at US$10 million.

Yet, the authoritative position Salma retained during her interactions with GAC workers at the start of this chapter reminds us that contrary to ideas about the purported dominance of Western aid organizations working in the global south, states and NGOs overlap and co-exist in complex ways. Global aid organizations, even the most prominent, well-funded ones, do not simply replace the state from below in what James Ferguson calls, "an imaginary topography of power." Rather they are configured more like, "horizontal contemporary organs of the state." As Ferguson explains, this means they are, "sometimes rivals, sometimes servants, sometimes watchdogs, and sometimes parasites, but in every case operating on the same level and in the same global space."[6] The meeting between Salma and GAC workers reflected this relationship, in which aid workers were alternately rivals and servants of the state, albeit situated in the global space of the aid organization. Thus, for instance, although Rana argued for a restructuring of police practices towards street children, she engaged Salma submissively. She might have openly contested her responses, like a rival who viewed the answers she received as insufficient, but she deferred to Salma as a powerful authority figure, a respectable woman, and an embodiment of the state.

Likewise, Salma retained an air of authority in all her engagements with the aid workers and even used a disciplinary, paternalistic tone when speaking to them, going so far as to point a finger at them in an attempt to silence their dissent. The authoritative practices Salma engaged in that morning, including paternal posturing and finger pointing, could not have been reversed and used against her by the aid workers in that same setting, even though workers retaliated against what they saw as her unsatisfactory responses. By carefully navigating the meeting as well as Salma's authority, the workers were situated within a horizontal state–NGO power structure. They were responsible for doing the work of the state, for transforming aspects of state governance that were at odds with international children's rights, but they remained configured "below" the state, as deferential subjects in roles that shifted, as Ferguson notes, between those of "rival and servant." Their interactions reveal a set of social relations that are far more complex than the typically imagined vertical state–NGO relationship, in which one exists below or above the other.

GAC workers were responsible for amending Egypt's Child Law, Code 126 (*Qanun al Tifl al Mu'addad*) using the language of children's rights and biomedical humanitarianism. Central to this was the inclusion of new categories into the law, which proved to be an ongoing point of contention for GAC workers, and not only in their face-to-face engagements with authority figures like Salma. They especially struggled to convey new ideas about childhood to groups such as Islamic leaders. New child-protection amendments based on international rights, as defined by the UNCRC, were contentious because they attempted to reconfigure definitions of the child itself, as well as the family unit, through notions of biomedical embodiment that emphasized individual autonomy over parental authority. In addition, they sought to expand state sovereignty into the domestic realm, deeming that state power took precedence over the authority of heads of households when it came to child welfare. This last point was most salient in the matter of "child abuse." Broadly, the new Child Law amendments sought to situate the state in stricter competition with parental authority on morally charged matters of the family, including child discipline and marriage.

New child-protection amendments also sought to dramatically shift relations between street children and police, redefining street children from criminal vagrants who threatened society's morality (*atfal mu'aradin lal-inhiraf*), into vulnerable children exposed to danger (*atfal mu'aradin lal-khatar*), the globally recognized category "children at risk." Thus, along with redefining the body of the child as autonomous and restructuring childhood in relation to the family, the new Child Law amendments GAC was promoting aimed to redefine how street children would be conceptualized in public—from would-be criminals who could be detained with adults as punishment to vulnerable children in need of compassion, rehabilitation, and humanitarian intervention.

A remarkable degree of human effort was required of GAC workers in order to accomplish these aims. They translated UNCRC information into Arabic for inclusion in the Child Law and then promoted the amendments through active, on the ground educational efforts in local communities. Subsequent to the Child Law's revision, GAC workers were expected to defer to state authorities relationally in face-to-face conversations while they educated them about international children's rights. This entailed awkwardly asserting knowledge about global rights, and reminding state authorities of their institution's own persistent violation of children, including the detention of children in adult facilities. Posters, flyers, and pamphlets circulated from global aid offices to key institutions such as schools, youth centers, and state ministries. These materials were geared towards teaching local populations that recognizing children's rights (*huquq al-tifl*) was natural and benevolent to children. As is the case with most children's rights discourse in Egypt, biomedical healthcare, and the right to health, was framed in this discourse as an integral part of international children's rights.

AMBIVALENT CONUNDRUMS: NAVIGATING A DOUBLE CONSCIOUSNESS AT WORK

When I interned at GAC, its main location was on the fourth floor of a massive office building situated in one of Cairo's most popular working-class neighborhoods. A major supermarket occupied the entire first floor of the building, providing GAC workers with a convenient pit stop on the way to or from work. When stepping out of the office building onto the largely unpaved streets, I was often faced with a string of vendors on either side of the building selling fruit, cigarettes, and packaged snacks. This centralized location in the heart of Cairo offered GAC workers easier access to important sites such as the offices of state ministries.

I spent my days at GAC helping to edit policy paperwork and assisting staff with simple office tasks such as making copies and translating legal documents. When I spoke with GAC workers throughout the day, as we completed our office tasks, they often commented about the "problems" inherent in children's rights, as well as the difficulties they were facing with their actual implementation in specific institutions, such as detention centers. In other words, they struggled with the gaps left open between global discourses and local realities. In her book *The Rise and Fall of Human Rights,* Lori Allen offers a compelling account of similar professional struggles. In documenting the deep cynicism that existed among human rights activists in Palestine—those who advocated for rights projects there—Allen calls attention to the "disdain and disregard" workers exhibited as they did their work while injustices persisted around them. Yet they continued to work for human rights despite their cynicism. They did so because they believed that they were, as Allen notes, "at least doing something against oppression, even if they knew that such work alone will not stop the abuses."[7]

Allen beautifully captures the deep sense of cynicism local rights activists experienced as they carried out projects in Palestine. GAC workers also shared cynicism about children's rights with me in this way, but far more frequently, they shared an all-encompassing sense of ambivalence towards their work. I define this ambivalence as a contradictory relationship they held towards their professional obligations as they related to international children's rights. In approaching their narratives through the analytic lens of ambivalence, rather than that of cynicism, as Allen has, I am capturing the dramatically polarized feelings they expressed about their work, including feelings of incredible hope, alongside utter disbelief, and their fighting for social justice initiatives despite an outright rejection of their very possibilities, of their actualization in real life.

As cultural intermediaries, GAC workers shared this sense of ambivalence along with a kind of "double consciousness." To have a double consciousness is to participate in two cultural spheres at once, in this case shifting between the global and local.[8] Having to negotiate two domains simultaneously in the office or at field sites such as state ministries or detention centers added to GAC work-related struggles. In my interviews, GAC workers conceptualized the domains of global vs. local through the categories of "Western ideas" and "Egyptian culture." Like the conundrums Merry identifies that arise from having to negotiate a double consciousness in order to implement international rights locally, GAC workers articulated a series of problems that the competing fields of "West" and "Egyptian" posed for them at work, for which they often had no resolution. These problems were most commonly identified as stagnant state bureaucracy, police oppression, Egyptian "culture," and a postcolonial relationship that situated Egypt in competition with, but always lagging behind, the West on matters concerning democracy and human rights. GAC workers pushed for child-centered reforms according to rights, but because of the "problems" noted above, they ultimately viewed their work goals as nearly impossible to achieve. For them, children's rights and Egyptian "culture" were inherently incompatible and on opposite ends of a spectrum when it came to child protection.

This conundrum—of pushing for reforms that may never actualize—reinforced an imagined global/local cultural divide for GAC workers in their professional lives. They spoke about themselves as situated firmly between the organization's main headquarters in London and the local Egyptian "culture" in which they were embedded and to which they belonged, but which stood against the tenets of child rights.[9] To them, they therefore occupied a liminal cultural position.

Workers viewed aspects of children's rights as far-fetched and impossible to implement in Egypt, but they still saw themselves as vital, educated experts who were doing morally just work in promoting rights. They articulated their professional goals as noble, in the sense that they were bringing children's rights "home" to places that needed reform, through grounded practices such as negotiations and translations. Yet even as they faced tenacious obstacles in their attempts to do this situated work, which often seemed impossible, they retained hope in the promises in children's rights discourse and in the possibility of establishing more equitable policies for children.[10]

In the next section, I delve deeper into the insights GAC aid workers shared with me regarding how they understood their professional roles and cultural liminality, as well as how they reframed global aid discourses into local vernacular.

IMPOSSIBLE SITUATIONS AND REWRITING EGYPT'S CHILD LAW

In 2008, GAC was constructing a massive countrywide strategy for the implementation of international children's rights in Egypt. One of its main goals, as I mentioned earlier, was to help revise Egypt's Child Law so that it would be more in line with UNCRC standards. Although the law was previously revised in 1996 to include some elements of international children's rights, key areas were left unchanged. As such, they posed problems for GAC and other global aid organizations in Egypt because they were incompatible with international humanitarian doctrines. Among these key areas was the legal age of marriage, which the law still fixed at sixteen. Other areas were the age of criminal responsibility, the definition of juvenile justice, notions of criminality related to child vagrancy and begging, and the absence of the category "child abuse" as a legally punishable violation. But in 2008, after nearly eight years of lobbying and political negotiation by GAC aid workers, and just as I was in the midst of my fieldwork with both CCI and GAC, the newly revised Child Law passed in parliament, bringing GAC's multi-year efforts to establish children's rights at home to a successful conclusion. But the months leading up to the law's passing proved arduous for GAC workers. Those who opposed the Child Law amendments made gripping headlines and conveyed compelling arguments against Westernization in the media that targeted an increasingly pious Muslim public. In response to the scathing press the new law was generating, GAC workers frantically collected data, drafted reports, crafted recommendations for government institutions, and consulted key figures like journalists and social activists. They hoped to counter the anti-Westernization arguments by promoting the revised Child Law as a pathway to social justice for vulnerable children and a means for the country to achieve progress.

One day, I walked into the GAC office to find workers gathered in a large conference room strategizing on how best to address public opposition and promote the new Child Law amendments. A conversation was under way about one of the most contentious amendments: the child-abuse clause. The inclusion of child abuse in the law generated some of the most caustic responses from local groups, for whom it most clearly represented a Western attempt to infiltrate and transform the very bedrock of "Egyptian culture"—the family, and specifically parental authority over children. Workers were discussing how to redefine the clause in campaign literature so as to protect children's bodily integrity yet remain attuned to the importance of Egyptian family values and especially parental authority. As the conversation progressed, workers seemed puzzled as to how to convey the notion that child abuse was inherently dangerous to the physical and emotional development of the child, so much so that it should constitute a crime punishable by law. Workers soon launched into a critique of "Egyptian culture," commenting on how ingrained physical punishment was in Egyptian child-rearing and how irreconcilable it was with children's rights.

The ways in which GAC workers described "culture" that day, as if it was in opposition to universal child rights, is actually a commonly held perception about rights, one dating back to the beginning of universal human rights itself. As anthropologists of human rights have noted, fears about the disappearance of local cultural difference in the face of global connections, such as international human rights, has been a core of post-eighteenth century European political philosophy and thinking.[11] Although these scholars contend that such an oppositional link, whereby a singular culture is pitted against universal rights, remains overly simplistic and obscures much of the diversity and debate that exists in specific places, the relationship reveals much about how particular groups negotiate and imagine the tensions that arise between global and local norms. Indeed, for GAC workers, the oppositional relationship between culture and children's rights, as it was articulated in office meetings and in the production of national policy, performed much ideological work. It reinforced workers' own sense of who they were in the continuous and ever-fluctuating process of bringing children's rights home.

As workers proceeded to complain about "Egyptian culture," 'Adil, the director and highest-ranking administrator in the office, interjected and reminded everyone that it was "their job" to change deeply engrained, traditional practices in the country. "This is going to be difficult," he remarked in an emphatic tone as everyone listened attentively, "but remember this is the *first time* [his emphasis] child abuse will ever be criminalized in Egyptian history!" His tone suddenly turned upbeat. He stood up in excitement and continued to encourage everyone in the room to keep pushing forward with the historic amendments because they signified a moral imperative, one that he said GAC aid workers were uniquely qualified to "bring" to Egypt.

'Adil's improvised speech was uplifting. It asserted that GAC workers were skilled experts and harbingers of rights. Moreover, it signaled that they were uniquely positioned to navigate the cultural space between GAC's London office and their home country. 'Adil's message to his staff was crystal-clear: only *you* can do this vital, momentous work. Motivational pep talks like this from 'Adil were common in the office when workers expressed reservations about tasks or complained about how untenable the premises of children's rights were in Egypt. In such moments of collective malaise and disbelief in the actualization of rights, 'Adil reasserted the historic role his office staff were playing. In meetings, he emphasized that creating a just, more equitable society was possible, but only through the arduous work that was taking place in offices such as theirs.

TEACHING RIGHTS TO STATE AUTHORITIES

There were several key areas of global aid work that engendered professional ambiguity for GAC workers and placed them between competing global and local forces. One area was education and outreach, which Rana performed regularly. Rana was one of the most prominent legal experts at GAC. She also considered herself a longtime human rights activist championing children's rights. At GAC she designed public outreach materials and pedagogical programs that sought to relay the core concepts of children's rights to state authorities as well as the general public. One of her professional goals was to ensure that the new Child Law would take hold in the state-run detention centers where street children were routinely held. To this end, she met regularly with state officials, conducted site visits, and cared for detained children, all in hopes of transforming how street children were perceived and handled by the state—transforming them from criminals to vulnerable victims. In all aspects of these responsibilities, Rana's work was gendered and relied on her performance of feminized characteristics, including mothering, nurturance, and the expression of emotions such as love and protection for the child. Doing this work required her to straddle various professional obligations based on her expertise and identity.

One afternoon I accompanied Rana to a state-run detention center, where she planned to meet with the manager of child-protection services in order to discourage security guards' use of physical force against street children. The center was located in a working-class neighborhood of Cairo, about thirty minutes' drive from GAC's office. The street children being held there were detained for anywhere from a day to several months. On the way to the center, as we sat through traffic and became increasingly more frustrated, Rana confessed that she hoped the face-to-face meeting with the manager would actually "do something" to change the way children were handled there. The confession revealed Rana's underlying fear that nothing, in fact, would change as a result of the visit, and her time would be wasted.

Driving up to the center, a massive cement structure heavily fenced off from the surrounding neighborhood by barbed wire, we had to pass a security checkpoint, where an armed guard inspected our car and then waved us in. After entering the center, another guard ushered us into a dimly lit office. The room was bare except for a plush leather sofa and wooden desk. Framed Islamic verses adorned the walls, conveying the manager's public religious piety. Soon after we settled onto the sofa the manager arrived and greeted us politely. Rana immediately began discussing GAC's campaign against "child abuse" as defined in children's rights. She explained to the manager that the new Child Law amendments meant that police had to change their handling of street children, and how acts that constituted physical or emotional abuse were criminalized under the new legal revisions. Rana then emphasized how the practice of handcuffing street children constituted a child-rights abuse under the new law. She urged the manager to convey this to guards and other state officials. Throughout the meeting, Rana maintained her professional demeanor and a respectful attitude, speaking to the manager in a polite, deferential tone just as she did with Salma during the meeting detailed at the start of this chapter. But her passion for the issues was evident. She begged the manager to consider the pain and trauma street children experienced in being transferred to detention centers. The manager listened patiently, sitting behind her desk with an aura of calm yet concerned authority. Like Salma's visit, this meeting illustrated how GAC workers were expected to educate state officials about international children's rights while remaining subordinate to them during face-to-face interactions.

Towards the end of the meeting, a security guard ushered two young boys into the room. Before our arrival, Rana had requested of the manager that she see children during the visit. As they entered the room, Rana stood up to greet them in a gentle, unthreatening manner. Placing a hand on one of their shoulders, she inspected their bodies and faces. She focused on the youngest boy, who appeared to be about eight years old. Sensing that he was the object of her inspection, he began inching his way, shyly, behind the security guard for protection. He had a deep scar running across his forehead, a sign that he had been "marked" as property by older boys on the streets.[12] The scar caught Rana's attention. She asked him questions about how long he had been on the streets and how the police had treated him. As he chewed nervously on a fingernail, he replied that he had left home because his father got drunk and hit him. Soon after he started living on the streets, a police officer had brought him to the center in handcuffs. This last bit of information reinforced Rana's desire to advise the manager on detention reform and police conduct with children. While the boy was narrating his story, Rana patted him on the back, indicating that she was a caregiver who meant him no harm. She also performed a disciplinary role during the interview, calmly directing the boy to speak when he took too long to answer. At one point, she commanded him to "take your finger out of your mouth when you speak." When he refused to respond in full, she demanded, "Answer the questions, OK?" In these ways, Rana re-inscribed her adult, maternal authority with the boy during the meeting. The entire interaction framed her as a mothering aid worker and professional figure employed by, and representative of, a global aid organization. Furthermore, the meeting served to override the manager's authority over children in the center by establishing Rana as the child's ultimate protector and caregiver.

In addition to the tensions these meetings created between Rana and state authorities, they provided Rana with evidence of children's bodily scars, wounds, and bruises. Seeing the violence up close and intimately on children's bodies fueled Rana's desire to push forward with national child rights reforms, despite the many challenges they posed in and outside of GAC offices. But even before working at GAC, Rana had considered herself a champion for social justice and vulnerable groups. After graduating from college, she began law school, but just before receiving her law degree, she dropped out to get married and start her own family. After giving birth to her second child, she felt ready to join the workforce and pursued administrative employment in GAC's legal department. She chose global aid work because it was a career that merged her passions for law, justice, and humanitarianism. In her office at GAC, she had a stack of playing cards that featured the face of the late Marxist revolutionary Che Guevara on her desk. This was simply one of the many ways in which she openly expressed her global citizenship and attachments to a cosmopolitan community of human rights advocates.

Rana was also a pious Sunni Muslim. She considered religious practices central to her identity, despite not veiling and always dressing in jeans, high heels, and colorful T-shirts for work. During the holy month of Ramadan, for instance, in keeping with proper notions of sacrifice and struggle, she fasted during daylight hours while sticking to her usual demanding work schedule. Her piety was not unusual, though it was more pronounced than that of other legal experts in the office. Workers at GAC were a mix of Coptic Christians, Sunni Muslims, and foreign expatriates, all of whom engaged in varying degrees of public religious practice. In the so-called secular space of the global aid office, workers generally observed religious holidays. In addition, the organization provided time off for anyone who requested it for that purpose.

At GAC, Rana's area of specialty was domestic child abuse. She was charged with overseeing the child-abuse amendment, the legal revision that she had the least faith in. She was most skeptical about how the amendment would take hold in real life and believed that the "average" Egyptian would simply disregard it. Rana cited her own identity as an Egyptian when making this claim, saying that her lifelong familiarity with Egyptian institutions and family politics supported her doubts. On the day when we received the news that parliament had passed the new child-abuse amendment, Rana was noticeably relieved and felt this justified the time and energy she had dedicated to the amendment. In a way, she felt her hard work had finally paid off, but she still felt skeptical about change taking hold on the ground. When I asked her why she was so doubtful the child-abuse amendment would initiate any observable change, she replied: "This amendment took forever, because for the first time in Egypt's history, the law interferes in domestic violence cases when a child is involved. It was difficult to implement this in the law because of this reason. It is because of our culture."

Seeking to better understand her response, I asked her to explain the difference between Egyptian culture and the culture reflected in the child-abuse amendment. Rana gave the question some thought, and then spoke of how families operated in Egypt. To her, it was radical for the state suddenly to intervene in family matters because a foreign organization deemed it necessary or correct. She emphasized how central child-rearing—cultivating the future—was to what it meant to be a good Egyptian, and that paternal authority would be undermined most by the child-abuse amendment. These were the reasons why revising the law was so arduous: "Before, parents, especially fathers, were the law in the family. From them, there was no place for children to turn to for protection from abuse. Now the law states that child abuse is a 'crime' and households are subject to intervention for the sake of the child. It took a lot of work to do this. It was a long process getting this done [changing the law]."

As this comment suggests, Rana believed the child-abuse amendment was historic, a change in the law that to some degree delegitimized the power of fathers over their own children—-a first for Egypt and a step towards a more just society for vulnerable children. In this respect, Rana expressed pride in her contributions to the amendment's successful passing. She saw this success as a professional achievement and a form of personal gain, being a long-time social justice advocate. By working to educate state authorities about children's rights, by translating global concepts into local law, and by promoting those new laws during face-to-face encounters, Rana, however, was constantly negotiating an ambiguous position as a cultural intermediary. She was constantly struggling to convey the tenets of children's rights locally, sharing a sense of hope in the possibilities that lay ahead for vulnerable children, notwithstanding her own doubts about the implementation of the law.

GLOBAL TENSIONS

Other aid workers at GAC saw the tensions in their work traverse national boundaries. They situated children's rights and medical aid for children within a broader global versus national relationship, and saw themselves as negotiating a transnational field of power, and not only local relationships, on behalf of vulnerable children. Magda was one such worker. She was an energetic twenty-four-year-old employee at GAC who echoed Rana's perspectives about the child-abuse amendment being nearly impossible to enforce in Egypt. Like Rana, she also emphasized how local family politics posed a major challenge to the new Child Law. Yet Magda often invoked a relationship between Egypt and the "West" in our conversations about her work at GAC. She saw Egypt lagging behind the developed world when it came to children's rights and broader issues of democracy and social justice, and she was deeply invested in both projects in and outside of her professional role at GAC.

Magda was the newest member of the office workforce when I was interning there. Despite being one of the youngest workers in the office, she was assigned a key, instrumental role in legal reforms because of her highly valued graduate education, multilingual skills, and professional research and writing experience. All of these factors were sought after in the global aid industry in Egypt. Magda was of Egyptian heritage, but had grown up in Paris. There, she attended reputable schools, where she mastered English while speaking Egyptian Arabic and French at home. Magda moved to London to complete her undergraduate studies and then earn a graduate degree in law, with a specialization in criminology. This transnational education, cultivated between Paris and London at two of the most respected institutions of higher learning, marked Magda as the ideal candidate for employment in GAC's legal department. Upon getting hired, she was immediately tasked with focusing on street children's health and protection and the other legal reforms GAC supported in the area of children's rights.

Magda's early childhood and adult life away from Cairo had not prevented her from developing a strong sense of Egyptian national identity. After receiving her graduate degree in London, Magda made the decision to move to Cairo specifically to work in the global aid industry. Her impulse, as she put it, was to "give back" to her country of origin. She felt she was uniquely qualified to contribute positively to Egyptian democracy and to legal reforms, because she saw herself as an expert in European political systems. Exposure to those systems, she believed, gave her insights that could improve policies in Egypt, her ultimate desire. Coming back home to Egypt meant a lot for Magda, she was once again, as she saw it, in touch with her "roots" and, at the same time, advancing a gratifying career in global aid at GAC. Giving back to Egypt, for Magda, meant fighting for social justice through any means necessary, whether it was in her global aid work or in her grass-roots political activism. While working at GAC, she also participated in protests and engaged in social activities on behalf of other vulnerable groups like women and prisoners. Magda was especially active in the mass demonstrations that swept the country in 2011 and 2013. We remained in touch after I completed this fieldwork, and she shared with me how she organized various meetings that led to marches and, from within her centrally located Cairo apartment, supplied protestors with water and safe spaces when they needed to hide from the security forces during the demonstrations.

One afternoon in the office just after the passage of the new Child Law, Magda reflected on the process. She was in high spirits. She felt the new law was a positive step for child welfare in the country. At the same time, she invoked the problem of global inequality when speaking about the law. Like Rana, she believed the new law would be impossible to implement in Egypt. She thought that the state was simply complying with the demands of more powerful states and not really invested in the protection of vulnerable children. Specifically, she talked about how Western-based aid institutions constantly applied pressure to countries in the Middle East like Egypt when it came to children's rights, explaining: "There's a reason why this is all taking effect now, at this moment in history. The reasons for these legal changes stem from international institutions like the UN applying pressure on Egypt to amend its laws."

Like Rana, Magda worked closely with state authority figures on the child-abuse amendment. She knew the official state narratives about children's rights quite well, and found them to be empty statements that served simply to improve Egypt's image abroad. In essence, the new Child Law would paint Egypt in a friendlier light in the eyes of Western states. It would appear as if it was on board with Western democratic ideals. Discussing global and national politics, Magda depicted the state as an actor that only "pretended" to care about children: "Because the government wants to have a good image abroad, especially when it comes to children, this [children's rights] is one of the things they want to pretend to have mastered."

Further elucidating the state's position on rights, Magda referred to local Islamists—the state's main political opposition. She noted that they contested the new Child Law because they saw it as an attack on Muslim identity and family morals, in which the West was oppressing Egypt by "planting the seeds of disunity between parents and children."[13] Magda understood this position despite not adhering to it herself. She cited a leading Islamic expert who described the child-abuse amendment as promoting the "sin of spying," because it would "encourage some people to interfere with the personal affairs of others, replacing compassion with hatred, and thus fragmenting society."[14] Attuned to these oppositional perspectives, Magda felt that it would be impossible to implement the new Child Law that had just passed. "It's a nice thought," she commented, "but in practice, it's very unrealistic." She went on to elaborate on what she believed were some of the practical problems that would prevent the child-abuse amendment from ever taking hold on the ground:

> In the [new] law, it says that anybody who knows that a child is in danger and doesn't refer them to the protection committee is liable for a fine. So, you, for example, know that your neighbor is hitting their child. You have to tell the protection committee. You are a teacher and you see another teach-

er mistreat a kid. You have to tell the committee. But the thing is, this is not enforceable. There is no specific obligation on people to do this, when you say this, it's just like saying, "Oh yeah, you know you have the obligation, otherwise you can be fined." But I mean who will enforce this? It's not practical. This in my opinion is one of the gaps in the law. When you say "everyone should tell," in the end, no one will.

As Magda's statement makes clear, the reporting of child abuse seemed impractical to her. In stipulating that "everyone should tell" if they witnessed child abuse, the law was too broad, and thus created a gap between itself and everyday practice. Moreover, Magda pointed to the lack of institutional accountability with respect to the law and the lack of police officers, social workers, or humanitarian workers to actually enforce such measures. She thus saw no resolution to the real-world problems associated with the child-abuse amendment.

Given the grim picture Magda painted, I asked her whether or not the new Child Law would do anything for vulnerable children in Egypt. Surprisingly, after expressing extreme cynicism about the amendments in previous statements, Magda shared how strongly she believed in the ideas put forth in the law. For her they were still, "a good thing for Egypt." The fact that new rights-based categories such as "children at risk" were included in the law gave Magda great hope and reflected a new "spirit" in the law with respect to children. This all signified better legal and ethical standings for street children, and that signified progress for Magda. Recalling shifts in how street children have been viewed in Egypt, Magda shared these thoughts:

I think it's better than what we had before [in the law]. Before, the spirit of the law was these kids are a social danger, so we will exclude them from society. This idea came from the 1950s and the social defense movement we had then. Now we have moved away from this view. It's more about rights. And you have to start somewhere. At least now they [the police] know they can't just put these kinds [of children] in the criminal justice system and have them arrested and detained with adults. That is counterproductive. I think it's a good step that we are getting away from this. Now we can address their needs and view them as vulnerable.

In Magda's account, the new Child Law was clearly a "good step" for Egypt. Its emphasis on the individual rights of the child and its framing of children as victims of bodily harm constituted an improvement in the way the state approached street children. Magda's belief that street children should be viewed as sufferers who arouse sympathy rather than criminals who require punishment points to their ascribed victim status in GAC policy, one that Didier Fassin discusses in other work on contemporary global humanitarianism.[15] Humanitarianism, according to Fassin's findings, re-categorizes subjects according to global knowledge and systems of classification. In this system, street children who are given the status of vulnerable (and helpless) victims not only excite sympathy, but merit compensation and new forms of intervention. For Magda, one area of compensation and intervention was safety from the police and a criminal justice system that imprisoned children with adults, where they could be physically and sexually abused.

Magda's perspectives about her work conveyed a sense that in Egypt things have improved for vulnerable children due to interventions by global aid organizations such as GAC, including major revisions to the Child Law. This work had the potential to reshape how children were approached by the police and society at large according to the model of the child in international children's rights. At the same time, Magda expressed great skepticism about the new rights-based amendments in the Child Law due to practical problems of enforcement, and did not think they would precipitate any real change on the ground. One day when we were discussing whether the perpetrators of child abuse would actually be convicted under the new law, and how the police would enforce the new child-abuse amendment, Magda giggled mischievously in the midst of our conversation and asked, "Who is ever going to report the officers who abuse the children? It's going to be the child's word against the officer's. And you know how that goes." Magda's sarcasm reflected her disbelief that a street child's word would be taken against that of an adult officer in state institutions. It illustrated an inescapable gap between the new Child Law and everyday life, one that GAC workers frequently struggled to reconcile as they pushed forward with reforms.

CULTURE AND THE STATE, PRESENT YET ABSENT

Other aid workers at GAC viewed Egyptian sociopolitical culture as the greatest obstacle to their professional goals. They spoke of the state as possessing a culture that was antithetical to children's rights, and narrated its relationship to GAC as one of presence yet absence. 'Adil expressed these views to me when we spoke about the new Child Law the day after it was passed. Like Magda and Rana, he was elated with the outcome but had much to say about the impossibility of key amendments, particularly the child-abuse amendment, actually taking hold in Egypt. 'Adil was most critical of the definition of "child abuse" in the law, and stated that local culture was in opposition to the concept as it was worded, saying:

> In Egypt, there are two actualities. First, abuse is widespread, common, and crosses all classes. Second, there's a problem with the definition of child abuse itself—there seems to be no concise definition of what child abuse is. There are few institutions equipped now to handle child-abuse cases in terms of protection, follow up, and criminalizing offenders. Yes, the problem of abuse exists, but it will be very difficult, culturally, to combat these issues, especially when it comes to entering people's homes and undermining the parents.

As 'Adil suggests, there were numerous problems associated with the child-abuse amendment that he struggled to resolve. One such problem was the widespread practice of physical abuse in Egypt—an issue that was rarely contested in the office. Most aid workers agreed that physical punishment was common in Egyptian households. But another problem for 'Adil was the lack of a working definition of "child abuse," one that could effectively be applied in state institutions to advance change. The third problem was that of state intervention itself, particularly when it came to the act of "entering people's homes" in child-abuse cases. In this respect, 'Adil expressed great doubts about the child-abuse amendment initiating intervention on behalf of children. He saw the state as powerful when it came to thwarting GAC initiatives, but absent in terms of advancing the law, given these intersecting problems. 'Adil's knowledge of the state—its various functions and bureaucratic processes—was extensive, and he often invoked the state in our interviews. He worked closely with state employees and was often the first point of contact between them and other GAC workers. Because of the frequency with which he dealt with state institutions, 'Adil's opinions about the state were well formed. He believed that "things got done" at a very slow pace at GAC because of the bureaucratic stagnation within governmental institutions.

In an ethnography of contemporary state bureaucracy in India, Akhil Gupta provides important insights into the affective and ideological work state narratives like these perform in everyday life.[16] As Gupta explains, narratives about the state imbue the state with a particular charisma and all-pervasiveness that both reproduce its power and reify its absence and illegitimacy. Narratives of the state also shape expectations of what the state can or cannot do, in this case, in the realm of global aid work. As Gupta notes and as 'Adil often showed me in the office, narratives about the state are "saturated with emotion," including humor, sarcasm, and irony as effective techniques for "coping with the absurdities of bureaucratic process."[17] I found 'Adil's daily comments about state inefficiency as important as big events like the dramatic meeting with Salma discussed at the start of this chapter.[18] Whether it was a quip about an unresponsive minister or an impromptu statement, shared in passing, about how much time it took to actually accomplish anything through formal channels, 'Adil's comments reflected the embattled relationship he had with the state. They illustrated how for him the state was all-encompassing in the workplace—imagined as always there—yet absent when it came to assistance in promoting GAC's policies and enforcing children's rights.

'Adil's unique perspectives were shaped by his demanding leadership position in a global aid organization. During the day, he was a top GAC administrator, overseeing all of the policy initiatives and staff across various departments. But in the evening, he was also a practicing physician with his own private practice. By retaining both professional positions, he managed to juggle two very demanding careers simultaneously—one in the global aid sector and the other in the private healthcare sector. He was also fluent in English, which allowed him to mediate effortlessly between authorities in GAC's London office and the staff in Cairo. When healthcare experts from London visited the Cairo office to conduct global health workshops, 'Adil was as an enthusiastic organizational liaison. He translated workshop presentations from English into Arabic for the staff members who were not bilingual and represented the needs of his staff when negotiating with foreign administrators. In this sense, 'Adil fully embodied the role of cultural intermediary at GAC, shifting from one linguistic sphere to another as he managed foreign professionals, local state authorities, and office staff.

CONCLUDING THOUGHTS

One afternoon as the workday ended, Magda and I decided to head to the supermarket on the first floor of GAC's office building for snacks. It was 4:00 p.m., the day had been long and full of tedious paperwork, and we needed a sugar fix. Earlier in the day, we had spoken about GAC's role in Egyptian governance. I had asked Magda if she could further explain GAC's relationship to the state, as she saw it. At the time, she confessed that she didn't have an adequate answer and would have to think about it. Now, as we negotiated the chocolate aisle in the supermarket under bright florescent lights, she turned to me and said, "Look, this is what the state does. When it comes to children's rights it has a tendency to just say 'Hey, NGOs, come and do it!' And you know what? The NGOs are doing it pretty well." Magda then seemed frustrated. She clearly felt that the state outsourced its duties to organizations like GAC and was not doing enough to protect children. She reiterated that NGOs like GAC were doing work for which the state was ultimately responsible. Wanting to know more about how she envisioned this discord, I asked, "So if the state is not doing this work and keeps delegating it to NGOs, then what *is* the state actually doing about children's rights?" Magda laughed out loud, once again, in sarcasm and shook her head. It was a laugh that I had come to recognize quite well in many of my conversations with GAC workers when I asked them about the bigger implications of their work, beyond the reports and grant documents they were producing that day. The response Magda then gave me reflected a sense of ambivalence regarding her place as a national subject working within a global aid industry. I sensed unease from her. She went on to elaborate:

> What does the state do? I don't know. Why don't you ask them? In the end, these kids should not be the responsibility of international organizations, because aid organizations are accountable to their funders, and [those] funders are not the state. So, how much does the state rely on aid organizations for children's rights? Actually, for everything. I don't think it's good, leaving everything to aid organizations. When it comes to this, the government doesn't do anything.

Magda's comment reiterated a key point elucidated in this chapter: that global aid workers are sometimes left in paradoxical positions, feeling ambivalent and even critical about their work. As Liisa Malkki has argued and similarly shown in research on Finnish humanitarians, aid workers can offer life-saving assistance in places of need, but they could also feel "ambivalent, inadequate, and even impure about the work they have done."[19] In mentioning that the state's outsourcing of child policy to aid organizations was not "good," Magda was doing more than simply criticizing the state. She was also positioning herself, as a global aid worker and an Egyptian social activist, in an ambiguous space, somewhere between being an agent and critic of global aid intervention. Her subjectivity also positioned her ambiguously, as a transnational expert who had lived in Europe for most of her life but was firmly grounded in an Egyptian national identity. Magda was deeply committed to her professional work at GAC and saw it as bleeding into her impulses for social justice activism beyond the office. Resembling a cultural intermediary, she translated knowledge between GAC London and Cairo, yet remained skeptical of the cultural logics behind aid policy. Moreover, she had lingering doubts about the overall efficacy of her work in practical, everyday life in Egypt. Magda's experiences and subjectivity were not unique in the global aid circles I observed in Cairo while conducting this research. Numerous global aid workers I encountered found themselves negotiating many of the same challenges, caught betwixt and between competing knowledge and practice, and wavering between hope and doubt in their efforts to craft transformational, rights-based policies on behalf of vulnerable children.

My time in GAC helped me better understand who the highly trained professionals who make global aid policy for Egypt are and what their sensibilities and personal attachments were. I became familiar with how they saw themselves in relation to their organization and society, as historical change-makers and as skilled cultural intermediaries, even if their goals were not accomplished. In particular, I witnessed how their labor practices included what they considered to be painstaking tasks, such as translating global knowledge, educating the public about international children's rights, and advocating for vulnerable children in the face of local state authorities. The professional roles these workers filled required that they be multilingual, educated (many were lawyers and doctors before working for GAC), and well versed in standard global aid doctrines—biomedicine and international children's rights—as well as their local cultures, societies, and histories. As I worked alongside GAC workers, I was struck with how often they attempted to manage and negotiate irreconcilable "frictions" associated with their work—grounded encounters that occur when global processes meet local realities. They engaged state authorities and oppositional groups persistently, and as best they could, drawing on the language of international children's rights and biomedicine to ultimately enact more humane and rights-based policies for children. Even after successfully passing new child-rights reforms, their everyday discourses reflected a mixture of optimism and disbelief in the actualization of those new doctrines.

Despite the many despairing comments that I documented in interviewing GAC workers about their roles aiding children—comments that called out ongoing inefficiencies and limitations at local levels—it was striking to me how they continued to imagine a society that would be safer, healthier, and more just for vulnerable children through their interventions. To this end, they considered the work they were engaged in at GAC a professional achievement and an ongoing and necessary personal struggle, even if it was riddled with challenges and disappointments. As legal and medical experts, they considered themselves working at the critical intersections between global and local forces, yet firmly rooted in a collective quest for greater social justice at home for vulnerable children.

CONCLUSION

THIS BOOK HAS BRIDGED THE CRITICAL STUDY OF GLOBAL MEDICAL aid with the cross-cultural study of childhood. My aim has been to offer readers a window into how global medical aid impacts individual children and local aid workers in contemporary Egypt—one of the world's most saturated global aid and development intervention hubs. Rather than an analysis of formal quantitative reports and statistics from above, I employed ethnographic methods to capture aid encounters *in practice*, as they took place in real time and among aid workers and child recipients. This intimate and grounded approach helps us understand what conventional reports and media headlines about aid with children cannot— namely, that global medical aid for children produces short and long-term effects that unsettle its unquestioned benevolence as a response to illness, suffering, and crisis. Above all else, the findings in this book challenge universal conceptualizations of the child in international children's rights and biomedical practice, respectively. The conclusions push us to contest the depoliticization and assumed passivity of children in global aid policy and during medical aid encounters. Instead, I suggest we view child medical aid recipients as subjects with the capacity to contest, reject, or reframe global medical action. For global aid organizations, the model of child in children's rights—the view that children are autonomous yet dependent on adults, rights-bearing yet without agency of their own and pure victims—has helped to promote healthcare, and biological intervention, as the ultimate panacea for childhood suffering in crisis zones around the world. Yet the

152   CONCLUSION

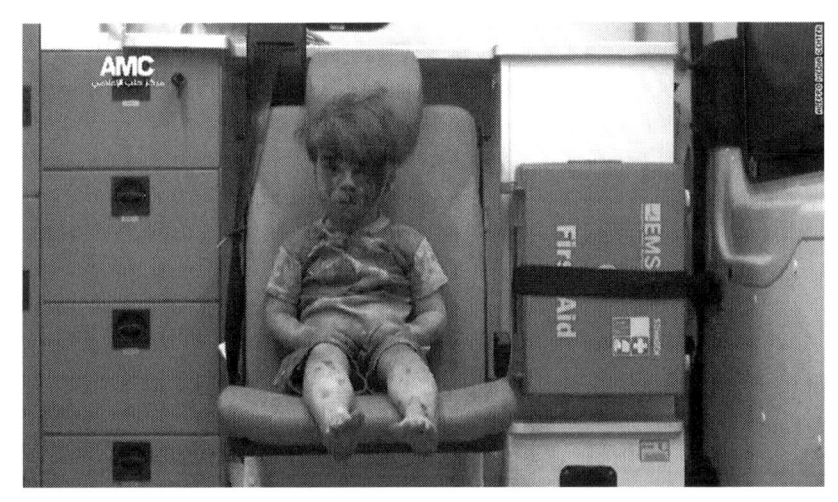

FIGURE 7. An image of Omran Daqneesh seated in an ambulance after being rescued from underneath rubble. Aleppo, Syria, June 2017. Source: CNN World, via Aleppo Media Center.

preceding chapters capture how street children and out-of-school village girls in Egypt, two key child recipient populations, negotiated medicine, met their own obligations, and strove to take care of themselves and others in the face of extreme adversity, at times in defiance of local aid workers.

Although this book focuses on a specific time and place, new global events challenge us to draw parallels and comparisons from the lessons I have learned about medical aid in Cairo. If we were unaware before the current novel coronavirus global pandemic that aid is precarious and paradoxical, these precarities and paradoxes have now been on full display worldwide since early January 2020. Medical aid workers and emergency healthcare personnel are political, economic, and social subjects, just like the people to whom they give care. They are subject to local, state, and federal bureaucratic structures, themselves filled with complexities and paradoxes. Imagine care for the homeless or vulnerable child patient in this context, even in seemingly developed environments such as the United States. Healthcare workers do not wait for state authorities or formal policy to attempt to save lives and to improvise care. In the United States, local governors struck deals with external agents, such as the government of South Korea, rather than wait for aid from their own president. Thus, there are many persistent themes from our experience of the current COVID-19 pandemic that were present throughout my research in Cairo from 2007 to 2009. Rather than the data in this book being viewed as particular to the so-called undeveloped global south or the crisis-riddled Middle East, the conditions that I studied and have documented might well be regarded as a harbinger of new ways of viewing emergency medical aid, ways that are worth urgent consideration by policy-makers and patients.[1]

My argument throughout has been that global medical aid is a paradox of care for children and aid workers in Egypt. For the children researched in this book, global medical aid represented an assemblage of material and social relations that produced contradictory outcomes. In addition to being a conduit of human compassion and care, aid was also a form of humanitarian governance, a mode of disciplinary power enacted upon young bodies and driven by the medical policies of global aid organizations. Such organizations operate through the neo-liberal state and aim to do its work, striving to heal, manage, and discipline vulnerable child populations in order to produce biomedically healthy, rights-bearing children. Interventions traced in this book range from shelter care to emergency mobile medical aid assistance, psychiatric care to protection from gendered child abuse. On the surface, all of this action ostensibly benefits the universal suffering child, wherever she may be, and speaks to the importance of upholding child bodily integrity in contexts of extreme poverty or crisis.

However, whatever their benefits, and there are many, global medical aid interventions were not culturally neutral, either in their conception or local execution. In the case of Egypt, they have reified, in policy, a range of gendered cultural stereotypes about poor children, rural communities, and Islam. For example, discourses about how local boys and men victimize village girls, a supposed symptom of their "traditional" or "Islamic" cultures, have found their way into global aid policy. These discourses were used to construct out-of-school village girls as victims of their communities and the worthiest of aid recipients in aid policy. As such they were critical to the advancement of the largest global village-girl youth project in Egypt's history. At the same time, dominant norms about gender, age, and class shaped how local aid workers distributed care to child aid recipients on the ground. The result was a gendered hierarchy of suffering among children that situated young girls at the top of the list of worthy sufferers and older, independent homeless boys at the very bottom. In some cases, these encounters with aid workers deepened homeless boys' pre-existing social marginalization, marking them as potential threats and "problems" in new, biomedical ways and in spaces such as children's shelters.

In sum, the global medical assistance children received from local aid workers was a paradox of care because it was both beneficial and limiting to them. It was useful when they sought urgent healthcare or other forms of support from aid workers, such as food, shelter, and friendship. It was limiting when workers restricted children's movement and practices, particularly when they wanted to work and make money and thereby manage their precarious economic conditions. For these children, gaining vital medical care from global aid organizations meant being intervened upon and regulated by local aid workers. Whether paid doctors or shelter volunteers, workers encouraged passivity and complacency from children during medical aid encounters, even if these efforts proved far from successful.

Inadvertently and otherwise, global medical aid policy aims to craft "healthy" childhoods around the world through aid interventions that draw from international children's rights and Western biomedical knowledge. Policy asserts that medical care is in the best interest of the child, community, and nation. Yet the street children and out-of-school village girls I came to know while working on this book routinely challenged, rejected, and struggled with the medical interventions they were subjected to. They also contested the disciplinary gaze of aid workers upon them, and understood assistance as a form of control, of governance. Rather than passively receive medical aid, these children renegotiated the terms of the biomedical encounter itself, or they avoided it altogether. Their experiences vividly illustrate the unanticipated gaps within global medical aid for children, and how global healthcare can fail to acknowledge, and in turn address, the political lives and needs of vulnerable children.

For local aid workers, medical aid for children was equally paradoxical as it created a specific set of benefits and limitations that shaped their professional practices. Workers gained valuable experience, prestige, and income as employees of prominent global aid organizations that operated transnationally. But they often struggled with how to distribute care and with their own inabilities to produce lasting, formally stated policy outcomes. Humanitarian doctors had to improvise their care-giving practices as best they could due to a range of roadblocks in their work environments. These roadblocks included children's medical noncompliance, stagnant national policies, limited humanitarian spaces and supplies, and local authorities who challenged the logic of rights, such as the police. As cultural intermediaries and medical experts situated between northern-based global aid offices, local institutional actors, and vulnerable child aid recipients, these workers often admitted to me that they had little faith in the long-term efficacy and success of their work. In other words, they did not believe they were making substantive changes in child health over the long run, mainly because they were not changing larger economic or political structures. Rather, most of them viewed themselves as participating in on-the-spot minimalist interventions, simply accepting that they just could not possibly do more.

At times, the despair of aid workers with respect to the limitations of their work, wide-scale poverty, and state repression was infectious and helped me view global medical aid as maintaining, rather than altering, the status quo for child aid recipients. Yet even with that deep-seated skepticism and despair, many aid workers also discussed their contributions in aid as an incredibly important ethical practice—they believed they were caregivers—and as potentially productive in other ways. For instance, many shared the sense that by assisting street children and village girls and by promoting new healthcare and child rights practices, they were contributing to a better imagined national future and to the phantasm of democracy in Egypt. Through that work, they believed they were in fact doing something for the social good, and beyond the Band-Aid provisioning of on-the-spot medical care.

These insights from both child recipients and aid workers fall outside the typical good/bad or success/failure binaries in terms of which we typically measure global health and medical aid outcomes. As such, they might be difficult for many people to accept, particularly because they do not provide clear-cut recommendations as to how we can effectively improve the lives of vulnerable children and ensure better futures. Even so, my observations with children in Egypt can, however, contribute to new perspectives and approaches to child suffering and vulnerability in aid. The first and perhaps most imperative of the perspectives I offer in this book is to approach child aid recipients as active, decision-making subjects and not as passive individual victims. This notion challenges long-standing constructs about child humanitarian recipients and their need for assistance. After all, medical humanitarian aid is meant for the most physically vulnerable in society, and who is more vulnerable than the child? The elevation of the child to the role of political subject or agentive social actor is contradictory to global aid constructions of those who are most in need. As such, it can also be counterintuitive to medical aid's overall goals, which is to save human lives. However, this approach opens new pathways for the creation of medical aid practices that confront, rather than elide, the performative practices and decision-making capacities of young recipients.

By far the most difficult aspect of writing this book has been my own grappling with the realities, present in each chapter, that vast amounts of resources and human labor are dedicated to medical aid projects for child aid recipients, yet these projects do little to fundamentally transform the underlying conditions that have harmed children's bodies and have kept them in a state of perpetual disenfranchisement. These interventions denied, or failed to center, children's political agency and their relations with the police. They eclipsed their ongoing need for money and their relationships with economic systems. The children I observed managed these conditions, just like other social groups around them. They did so while drawing upon and renegotiating medical and social resources provided by global aid organizations. In some instances, their young and gendered status exposed them to more discipline and violence than other groups. This was the case with street boys who were objects of police aggression and who utilized a mobile clinic for social solidarity and safety, as well as medical care.

Despite the complex realities that I have outlined throughout this book, global aid organizations operating in Egypt and elsewhere in the Middle East continue to approach children as apolitical recipients of care and as de facto compliant biomedical subjects. In global medical policy for the region, they appear voiceless and victimized by local circumstances. Major corporate donors—from ExxonMobil to Nike—reinforce this model of childhood vulnerability for the obvious reasons. It is a model based on international children's rights and middle-class notions of family and domesticity. It neatly and universally infantilizes children in faraway places and situates them outside of history and culture. This book demonstrates how this model of childhood inaccurately represents the lived experiences of child aid recipients in Egypt. More importantly, the model has the potential to harm children by deepening their social marginalization, stripping them of voice, and eclipsing the structural violence they and others routinely endure every day. And as violence is eclipsed in policy, so are the creative resistance strategies children must employ to keep their bodies safe and to stay alive.

In light of this, it is clear that global health and medical aid industries, as well as the donors who provide their funding and sustain their work, must radically shift their approach to children to one that recognizes, and legitimates, their bodily suffering alongside their social suffering and political constitution.[2]

THE ARAB SPRING: SEEING THE CHILD IN EGYPT AS A POLITICAL SUBJECT

Whereas global aid organizations deny or eclipse children's political constitution in their policies, local populations and states can recognized them—albeit in differing ways and during different historical moments—as political and economic actors, as national subjects with the potential for patriotism and martyrdom, and as powerful subjects who may be threatening to adults or society at large. Scholars, especially historians, of modern Egypt have presented us with diverse accounts of childhood that contest the validity and universality of the figure of the child in international children's rights and global medical aid policy.[3] These studies point to conceptualizations of young people that politicize them. Rather than romanticize the life phase of childhood as a distinct phase in the human life cycle and the child as passive and dependent, these works emphasize children as socioeconomic actors with political life-worlds that are enmeshed in those of adults, through labor, large extended families, communities, and religion.[4] Taking us back to the nineteenth and early twentieth centuries, when Egypt underwent a period of rapid modernization and anti-imperial struggle, these studies suggest that the life-worlds of Egyptian children have always been riddled with national politics, and those political realities shaped children's practices and subjectivities.[5]

One recent iteration of a more diverse approach to childhood in Egypt, one that recognizes children as political subjects, emerged from the Arab Spring, the anti-government mass uprisings that swept through the Middle East and North Africa in 2011 and permanently transformed the region in ways that have both opened up and foreclosed democratic possibilities for citizens. In research on the revolutionary uprisings in Egypt, Chiara Diana has focused on street children's active roles during the public protests. Like adults, street children protested and even died at the hands of government security forces. Subsequently, fellow citizens ascribed to them the status of martyrs of the Egyptian revolution.[6] As Diana notes, the ways in which Egyptians hailed killed street children as national martyrs rendered the boundaries between childhood and adulthood permeable and less distinct, and ascribed onto children a degree of political agency that is absent in global aid policy.

The category of the child martyr—the figure that sacrifices life for nation—helps us grasp how children in Egypt could be viewed as both vulnerable subjects and as political agents embedded in social relationships; as marginal victims of militarized state power and as decision-making subjects who have the capacity to protest government policies. Like the street children who lived at CCI's homeless children's shelter, or the boys who used the organization's mobile medical clinic (chapters 1 and 2), child martyrs of the Egyptian revolution used their bodies in public space as a rhetorical device, as a vehicle for emancipation in the face of governmental power. But unlike the adults who protested during the demonstrations, their homeless bodies—constantly visible in public spaces—symbolized the very poverty that protestors were condemning. These children, as Diana suggests, occupied a key role during the mass uprisings in Egypt. Despite their vulnerable youthful status, they were still viewed to have fought "for the people" in ways similar to adults.[7]

The events that I observed in this book occurred only months before the Arab Spring took hold across the region in 2011. In the winter of 2012, as Egypt was transitioning into a new presidency, I returned to Cairo for a follow-up visit. I was hoping to learn how the demonstrations had affected my research interlocutors and everyday life for Egyptians. At the time, roughly a year had passed since the first demonstrations took place in Egypt. For eighteen dramatic days, Egyptians across the social spectrum—young and old, poor and well to do—flooded Tahrir Square in Cairo in an act of anti-state defiance. As the world looked on, they demanded jobs, healthcare, and an end to decades of authoritarian state repression. After nearly a thousand deaths at the hands of state police, the protestors—steadfast in their call for social justice and human dignity—successfully ousted the now late president Hosni Mubarak. Many decreed the explosive events a "revolution," because, for the first time in Egypt's modern history, a leader had been deposed through popular revolt and through the extraordinary will of the people. Others asserted that while the head of the state had been ousted, an entrenched and recalcitrant state, a postcolonial authoritarian regime propped up by Western powers, remained intact. For them it would require deep structural transformations, far more than simply removing a political figurehead, to enact regime change in the country.[8] The aid workers in this book held both views about the revolutionary events as they described this transitional phase to me.

A few days after landing in Cairo, I met with Magda (see chapter 5). Over coffee in a downtown café, she talked about how she had resigned from her position in GAC a few months after I departed Egypt. She had secured a job in the legal department of a smaller, locally run human rights NGO. She was passionate about this new job and believed it allowed her to defend the human rights of all Egyptians in a more direct manner. The democratically elected Muslim Brotherhood–related

Mohamed Morsi was now president and Magda's dreams of a more just, post-revolutionary society seemed lost. As she described it to me, she watched the new president initiate intensive crack-downs on human rights activists and grass-roots NGOs like the one she was working for. Moreover, as she put it, Morsi was aiming to consolidate power by revising the constitution and stifling anti–Muslim Brotherhood opposition, thereby further empowering the state. Magda appeared more anxious and worried than ever before as she described the recent events. "We've been through a lot this last year," she recounted, sharing how she housed and fed protesters in her downtown apartment during the demonstrations. Her hands shook as she sipped coffee and spoke about the terror and exhilaration she had felt while protesting in Tahrir Square. She predicted that more social instability, more violence, was to come, and she was right.

In 2012, widespread opposition against Morsi led to more waves of public protests across the country, accompanied by more violence, and more deaths by government forces. As a result, a new president, this time an army general from Mubarak's previous regime named Abdel Fattah el-Sisi, took power in July 2013. At the time of this writing, he remains president. To date, his legacy has been marked by strong ties to Mubarak's pre-revolution regime, an increase in support from Western powers, and a rise in repressive tactics against Egyptian citizens calling for democratic freedom, particularly journalists, academics, and other public regime critics.

Throughout these turbulent transformations in Egypt's recent history, children remained at the center of national discourse. Returning to the discussion of street children as martyrs, during the first mass uprisings in Cairo, we witnessed how street children put their physical bodies on the line during public protests. They marched, lifted banners, and were among the first to be shot during the initial days of the uprisings. Local news reports produced during that time described street children as Egypt's "smallest soldiers," those who braved tear gas, bullets, and beatings alongside other protesters in their quest for human dignity.[9] Even international media painted street children as the one social group that was "forever abused by the regime" and "a living condemnation" of it.[10] Rather than infantilize the vulnerable child, these depictions used the child's suffering body as a metaphor for the suffering nation. They elicited compassion for the child who was encountering state violence, but they also enmeshed the child subject in webs of social, cultural, and political relations, all while granting children a sense of agency and decision-making power.[11]

BRINGING SOCIAL JUSTICE INTO GLOBAL MEDICAL ACTION

The findings in this book encourage new questions around how we can conceptualize children's suffering and, in turn, reimagine care. If global intervention remains on the rise, is it possible for aid organizations to employ a more expansive, diverse model of childhood? What would medical aid policy look like if it drew upon more expansive notions of childhood suffering, notions that include social justice? I believe we can begin to answer these questions by first seeking to understand children's full experiences with global medical aid in specific places, which entails exploring how they view their bodies in relation to medical assistance, and why they may or may not resist adult care. Global medical aid has life-saving potential for children, as we know, but a central argument of this book maintains that it does not address children's long-term needs for collective social justice and political-economic equity—conditions that become biological realities for children. Medical aid policy claims to protect and heal child bodies, yet it does not provide the kind of universal care required to improve human well-being in the long run. How can a single child body remain healthy when society at large is sick? Wouldn't the broader sicknesses eventually infect the individual child body? Global medical aid policy constructs child bodies as autonomous, undeveloped, and passive. This physically wounded, apolitical child is recognized as worthy of compassion and care, heralded as part of a universal child humanity driven by international children's rights. In policy, as I have mentioned, such a child does not resemble a laboring and politically exploited child entangled in social relations.[12]

One key paradox inherent to global medical aid is that sicknesses lie in broader societies as well as individual human bodies. If that social suffering is not addressed, vulnerable children remain sick, wounded, and unsafe. I have sought to convey in this ethnography that children themselves know this. As child aid recipients negotiate vital biomedicine in the absence of other forms of care, the interventions remain limited. Moreover, they are driven by a set of cultural assumptions about the Middle East that eclipse or even exacerbate global and local inequalities (see chapter 4). The children throughout this book contest those assumptions in their confrontations with the state, rejection of biomedicine, and continued participation in labor markets. These experiences deserve recognition and legitimacy in global humanitarian industries, not only children's passive and dependent status.

Once we understand children's full experiences with global medical aid, as I have sought to do in this book, we can begin to ask a different set of questions about their vulnerability. For instance, how do children manage their own bodies in the absence of adult care? How do they strive to secure safety and social justice in their own names? Along with a need for biological health, the answers to these questions can foreground children's social experiences and culturally constituted lives. They would help aid organizations craft a language of physical suffering that deinfantilizes childhood and illuminates a broader landscape of political crisis. At the same time, they would shine a light on social suffering alongside biological suffering in local contexts. To do so would bring us closer towards the forces (global and national) that produced suffering in the first place.

BEYOND REPRESENTATIONS OF CHILDHOOD BODILY SUFFERING

Today, as crises rage on in the Middle East, global aid organizations continue to describe the region as a volatile humanitarian disaster zone. This volatility is attributed to ongoing political upheavals occurring in Syria, Iraq, Yemen, Gaza, and Afghanistan, and to the refugees that continue to flow into neighboring countries and European border zones as a result. In addition to these humanitarian disasters, at the time of this writing the coronavirus pandemic has taken hold in the region—a historic event that has deepened the vulnerability of aid recipient groups and situated medical workers on the front lines of multiple, interconnected crises. The aid discourses that are likely to emerge in the coming years about the region will continue to identify child bodies as the most vulnerable of their societies. They will increasingly represent the Middle Eastern child—through various media images and policy channels—as lacking any individual agency and lying outside of local culture and politics.

This book has argued that such depictions of childhood suffering are problematic and worthy of sustained critique beyond aid industries. The complex experiences street children and village girls had with biomedical care described in the preceding chapters demonstrate that we need to interrogate the ways in which their bodies were put to use by global aid organizations. Representations of Middle Eastern children's suffering produce value for aid industries. Beyond organizations, I suggest we ask what consequences those representations of the body produce for local populations and for children themselves.

Arthur and Joan Kleinman have compelling arguments related to the cultural appropriation of suffering in global humanitarian industries. They urge us to explore, both morally and politically, how images are used to further humanitarian responses to disasters.[13] Suffering is neither universal nor essential, and there is no single way in which humans suffer. Yet they point out that vulnerable African children are typically depicted in Western images alone, unaccompanied by other local people. This suggests that their suffering is an isolated experience rather than a collective and social one. The remedy or intervention, as the assumptions purport, must then also be individualized and targeting the child, not the community or the reform of national and regional policies. Worse still, local communities and governments appear incompetent, irrational, or destructive in these depictions of lone suffering children. Such practices of cultural appropriation almost always paint the West as "better" and more "civilized" than African societies.[14] Such is the paternalistic and powerful position global aid organizations hold in media from afar.

Paradoxes of Care offers a different story about the power of global aid organizations on the ground in Egypt. Local aid workers employed by American and European-based global aid organizations translated knowledge for organizations and put medical aid policy into practice through their various struggles, successes, and improvisations with child recipients and local authorities. As demonstrated in chapter 5, these processes were far from seamless and singular. They were fraught with friction and ambivalences, and they challenged the dominant view that global aid organizations travel around the world to effortlessly penetrate local states in crisis in their quest to help children. Their power and paternalism was contested by the aid workers in this book.

Global aid organizations nevertheless have extraordinary representational power over how children are depicted in global aid policy and media. In the wake of numerous contemporary humanitarian disasters, Middle Eastern children have been depicted as suffering alone and independent of local communities, just as Kleinman and Kleinman have shown for the African child. This professional practice is common beyond aid industries. We may recall how in 2017 the bloodied face of young Omran Daqneesh, a Syrian boy from Aleppo who was pulled from rubble after a government airstrike, shook the world when his image circulated in mass media outlets. The image initiated international public outcry against the violence of the Syrian Civil War like no other.[15] At the time of the story, the crisis was in its fifth year, and thousands had already lost their lives, while millions had been internally and externally displaced. In media articles, Omran was routinely described as an "innocent" child who was "in shock" and traumatized. His dusty face and tiny body directly faced the camera in each image, while captions described him as a representation of the entire war. One article even labeled him the symbol of Syrian national suffering.[16]

CONCLUSION 163

Omran was not the only local child to have elicited global compassion on a scale this wide and to have been featured alone, suffering. Alan Kurdi's lifeless three-year old body washed ashore on a Turkish beach in 2015. Images quickly circulated featuring him lying face down in the sand with his shoes still on. More than the subsequent images that featured his bereaved father, the image of Alan alone in the sand became the symbol of Syrian suffering. It was used to condemn the ongoing crisis and win support for refugees and migrants who endured the deadly journey at sea each day.[17]

In 2018, I spoke with a Syrian physician about his medical relief work during the Syrian war and mentioned the wide-scale attention young Omran had garnered in the media. This aid worker was quick to point out that Omran's image was partial in that it did not capture significant aspects of the social context in which it was taken. Then, he surprised me by calling Omran, "one of the lucky ones." After witnessing countless deaths through his global medical aid work, this doctor considered Omran fortunate, because he was rescued from the rubble and was able to live. "So many other children," he stressed, "died in those airstrikes. But Omran lived, and has a family." What was categorically missing from Omran's famous media image, he stressed, were his siblings, parents, and other Syrians who were not so lucky. They perished under the rubble during that same aerial bombing.

This doctor's view of young Omran differed widely from the descriptions about him in media articles. Rather than viewing Omran as a lone traumatized child, he viewed him as lucky, embedded in a family, and bound to broader political struggles. Humanitarian aid organizations, however, depict children in their policies just as the mainstream media does when they portray distant disasters—as individual and voiceless embodiments of crisis. Such naturalized depictions are powerful and valuable for aid industries. They incite compassion among publics and propel streams of donor funding for humanitarian causes. As McKenzie Wark has noted, when we consume such images, we "cannot help but feel something."[18] Those feelings lead to moral outrage, and then to immediate action, all in the name of the suffering child.

But other conceptualizations of suffering can situate children both within their local worlds and at the same time in interconnected social, political, and economic realities. These better models of childhood, like the one offered by the Syrian aid worker I discussed above, bring distant and obscure humanitarian disasters into sharper, more complex focus, following Kleinman and Kleinman. If anything, they shed light on the full scale of collective trauma in the region and the political underpinnings of suffering. Unlike the model of the child in children's rights, the models I propose mark children as social rather than individual sufferers in aid. Responses and support can then shift from a sole focus on individual children, or biological health, to the sources of collective pain, illness, and death.

The children at the heart of this book convey an urgent need for a revision of the model of the child in global medical aid policy and in popular images of the Middle East along these lines. Their stories remind us that treating the bodies of individual children is not enough. Suffering is at once biological and social. By negotiating care and reframing the humanitarian encounter, these children illustrate the promises and perils of medical action driven by rights. Their need for social justice reshapes how we conceive of global aid, as well as the politics of childhood and healthcare.

Notes

INTRODUCTION

1. I am indebted to Geneviève Negrón-Gonzales's powerful chapter, "Teaching Poverty," in Roy et al. 2016 for opening up this conversation and shaping my thoughts on media, humanitarianism, and poverty.

2. For more on the unintended consequences of international aid for suffering children, particularly in the case of postcolonial Africa, see Bornstein 2005 and Dahl 2014 and 2015.

3. This campaign can be accessed by visiting www.girlup.org.

4. Abramowitz and Panter-Brick 2015; Bornstein 2005; Cabot 2016; Dubal 2018; Ferguson 1994.

5. Caldron et al. 2016.

6. Lotfi 2018.

7. Bornstein and Redfield 2010: 6.

8. James 2010; Ticktin 2011: 16.

9. See also Sanford and Carter 2020 on the subject of race, class, and pandemics. They argue that the Spanish Flu impacted African Americans in St. Louis at higher rates due to failing infrastructure and unequal access to public healthcare. As they accurately point out, pandemics are not great "equalizers," but rather forces that devastate the most vulnerable populations the most, thereby exacerbating preexisting social disparities.

10. Biehl and Petryna 2013

11. Vaughan 1991.

12. In this book, I have attempted to adopt Kristen Cheney's (2011) approach to ethnographic research with children, which allows children to guide and participate in research alongside the ethnographer. In this way, children are granted agency and power within the research process as knowledge is produced about them.

13. Roy 2010.

14. George Marcus (1995) writes about the importance of multi-sited ethnography in our contemporary globalized moment. Marcus argues that an increasingly globalized world calls for new ethnographic methods that focus less on space and more on connection, networks, and movement.

15. Bluebond-Langner and Korbin 2008; Allerton 2018.

16. Hunleth 2013.

17. Rose 2006; Feldman and Ticktin 2010: 16–17.

18. Cole and Durham 2007 also focus on children as key objects and drivers of globalization.

19. Fassin 2012; Feldman and Ticktin 2010.

20. Dewachi 2015.

21. Here I am extending the influential findings of the anthropologist Julie Livingston (2012: 6) who has demonstrated that improvisation is a defining feature of biomedicine in Africa. Livingston, who conducted ethnographic research in an oncology ward, approaches biomedicine as a global system of knowledge and practice that is also highly contextualized and contingent on the labor of particular people.

22. Fassin 2013 elucidates the subject of global "hierarchies of suffering" in aid for children in Africa. In a study on HIV/AIDS in South Africa, Fassin found that there was a moral hierarchy of sufferers in international humanitarianism. At the top of this hierarchy were the seemingly blameless, purely innocent children, while their parents were situated below, as undisciplined subjects who were incapable of assisting them. These moralizing representations of African kinship reflect Western imaginaries about Africa and African sexuality. Fassin reveals how these racialized, stereotypical representations make their way into public health policy and justify continued intervention on behalf of children.

23. McKay 2018: 12.

24. These findings were present in a UNICEF Middle East and North Africa Report published in 2019.

25. Malkki 2015: 7.

26. Feldman 2008.

27. Herrera and Bayat 2010; Said 1979.

28. Roy 2010: 16.

29. Singerman and Amar 2006.

30. These findings were present in a UNICEF Middle East and North Africa Appeal titled "Humanitarian Action for Children," published in 2018.

31. Wendland 2010.

32. Ong 2006; Sassen 2001; Winegar 2006.

33. Amar 2013; El-Shewy 2013; Comaroff and Comaroff 2000; Harvey 2006.

34. Elyachar 2005; Ferguson 2006.

35. McKay 2012.

36. Beinin 2005; Henry and Springborg 2010; A. G. Marshall 2013.

37. Altorki and El-Solh 1988; Geertz 1977.

CHAPTER 1

1. Ferguson 1994.

2. For more on the structured nature and seriousness of children's play across cultures, see Schwartzman 2011 [1978].

3. Bhabha 2005.

4. Honwana and de Boeck 2005; Stephens 1995.

5. Cole and Durham 2007; Honwana and de Boeck 2005; Stephens 1995.

6. Samaan 2008.

7. Asad 2000; Malkki 2015; Cheney 2007; Malkki and Martin 2003; Montgomery 2009; Scheper-Hughes and Sargent 1998; Shepler 2005; Stephens 1995.

8. Scheper-Hughes and Hoffman 1998.

9. Montgomery 2001: 83.

10. Honwana and de Boeck 2005.

11. Sinervo 2013.

CHAPTER 2

1. In Cairo, community pharmacies can also serve as informal healthcare centers. If requested to, pharmacists sometimes for a fee deliver quick emergency medical care by treating minor wounds, infections, or ailments on the spot.

2. In ethnographies about ethics and Egyptian healthcare, Sherine Hamdy (2008; 2012) discusses the failures of the state when it comes to providing adequate care to Egypt's poor and working classes. Hamdy details how Egyptians must resort to

other, informal and private, healthcare assemblages in order to manage the gaps and deficiencies in state-sponsored public healthcare.

3. For more on how global humanitarianism with children produces unintended social effects, see the work of the anthropologist Bianca Dahl (2009; 2014; 2015).

4. Ghannam 2013: 5.

5. Kleinman 1988.

6. See especially Redfield 2013: 73–74 for more on this extensive history of mobile medicine, particularly with respect to Médecins Sans Frontières.

7. Ibid., 71.

8. See, e.g., "Mobile Health Teams Help Save Children's Lives in Yemen" (Sanaa, September 28, 2016), www.unicef.org/yemen/press-releases/mobile-health-teams-help-save-childrens-lives-yemen-unicef.

9. Mauss 2000 [1925].

10. In a classic essay, Louis Althusser (1971) presents the concept of "hailing" as a means through which the concrete subject is identified by the state apparatus and produced. I use the term here to denote how the humanitarian mobile clinic, in a somewhat similar fashion, aimed to produce a particular kind of child and imposed subjectivity through its actions of gift-giving and education.

11. For more on humanitarian biopolitical governance, see Feldman and Ticktin 2010; Ong 2006; Rose 2006.

12. Redfield 2013: 88.

13. Ibid.

14. Gordon 1988.

15. Feldman 2018: 98–99.

16. From Malkki 2015 as referenced in Feldman 2018: 99.

17. See also Honwana and de Boeck 2005, 32–38, on child soldiers, who similarly evoke social anxiety and international humanitarian concern. Much like street children, child soldiers upset social norms of children's innocence and dependency, turning the world upside down.

18. Hunleth 2017.

19. Kleinman 1988: 8–15.

20. Cox 2015.

21. For more on the concept of "social wounds" in contrast to individual wounds and resulting from political forces, see Dewachi 2015.

22. Inhorn 2003 is particularly informative here in an ethnography detailing how underserved or illiterate women in Egypt access global biomedical knowledge and

healthcare. Inhorn focuses on class disparities in Egypt, revealing how when it comes to formal healthcare, such women are left out of global science's so-called emancipatory and democratic potential.

23. O'Neill 2014 explores the intricate and lasting traumas to the body associated with homelessness in ethnographic work on post-communist Bucharest.

24. Redfield 2013: 90.

25. Cabot 2016.

26. Amar 2016.

CHAPTER 3

1. Portions of this chapter were previously published in slightly different form in Sweis 2017c, "Security and the Traumatized Street Child: How Gender Shapes International Psychiatric Aid in Cairo," *Medical Anthropology Quarterly* 32 (1): 5–21.

2. David Marshall (2014) has discovered similar results in a study of international psycho-social assistance and trauma care among Palestinian children. Here, the traumatized Palestinian child is constructed as both a victim and a threat through such interventions. My research also emphasizes how this threatening status is unequally applied to boys, and therefore gendered.

3. Fassin and Rechtman 2009: 4.

4. Ibid.

5. Wark 1995.

6. Ibid., 10.

7. Caldeira 2000; Honwana and de Boeck 2005; O'Neill 2014; Shepler 2005; Simone 2004.

8. Metzl 2009: xi–xiv.

9. Feldman 2008; Ticktin 2006.

10. Ticktin 2011.

11. Martin 2007.

12. Foucault 1977.

13. As Farha Ghannam (2013: 32–33) argues, poor and working-class boys in Cairo must develop certain markers of masculinity in order to succeed in making money and maintaining relationships as masculine subjects. She writes that boys struggle to embody the materialization of toughness and strength. They must do so while remaining under the watchful gaze of others. This is how they assert their subjectivity and social standing as a "man."

14. Gupta 2012.

15. Kleinman 1988.

16. Mattingly 2010: 108.

17. A study by Okuma (1983) revealed how within North American psychiatry, Tegretol and other carbamazepines are best known for having therapeutic and prophylactic effects on bipolar disorders.

18. Dumit 2012.

19. LeFrancois 2007 and 2013.

20. Hecht 1998: 24.

CHAPTER 4

1. Portions of this chapter were published in slightly different form in Sweis 2012 "Saving Egypt's Village Girls: Humanity, Rights, and Gendered Vulnerability in a Global Youth Initiative," *Journal of Middle East Women's Studies* 8, no. 2 (2012):26–50. Sections were also published in the chapter "Do Muslim Village Girls Need Saving? Critical Reflections on Gender and Childhood Suffering in International Aid," in *The Global Status of Women and Girls: A Multidisciplinary Approach*, edited by Lori Underwood and Dawn Hutchinson (Lanham, MD: Lexington Books, 2017). All rights reserved.

2. Fassin 2010.

3. Ali and Minoui 2010.

4. Ibid., 10.

5. Ibid.

6. Chatterjee 1989: 623.

7. Sweis 2012: 26–50.

8. As mentioned in the Introduction, the UN Foundation's Girl Up initiative is one such project. Launched in 2010, it aimed to empower girls worldwide in their fight against gender inequity. Girls in the global north were "hailed" (cf. Althusser 1971) through various online campaigns as key participants who could empower village girls across the global south through a shared girlhood status.

9. Abu-Lughod 2013: 143.

10. Chatterjee 1989: 623.

11. Ahmed 1992.

12. Mahmood 2005.

13. Mohanty 1988: 72.

14. Ibid., 79.

15. Malkki 2015.

16. Ibid., 77.

17. Data from the World Bank, 2018.

18. Ali 2002.

19. See Population Council, "The Ishraq Program in Rural Upper Egypt" (2006), 4, www.sportanddev.org/sites/default/files/downloads/66__providing_new_opportunities_to_adolescent_girls_in_socially_conservative_settings.pdf.

20. Malkki 2015: 95–98.

21. Mitchell 2002: 153–78.

22. Chatterjee 1989. See also Lockman 1994 on the discursive dimensions of national class formation and identity among Egyptian intellectuals and the working class around the turn of the century.

23. As in rural Egypt, girls in Zambia also face substantial gender-based challenges in reconciling school and household responsibilities. See Hunleth et al. 2015.

24. See further Hengeveld 2015.

25. Malkki 2015.

26. Ibid.

27. Ibid., 8.

CHAPTER 5

1. Tsing 2005: 1–10.

2. Omidian and Panter-Brick 2015.

3. Citing political theorists, Amal Hassan Fadlalla (2018: 15) uses the terms "global citizenship" and "cosmopolitan citizens" to describe a transnational community that binds people together through a desire for social justice and human rights. Similarly, workers at GAC saw themselves as belonging to a transnational community of global citizens who promoted human rights.

4. Mitchell 2002.

5. Merry 2006.

6. Ferguson 2006: 103.

7. Allen 2013: 20.

8. Ibid.

9. On the subject of the culture concept in the Middle East, Winegar and Bishara (2009) take note of the various complexities associated with the uses of culture by local elites and activists. They argue that while within anthropology the concept has been rightfully critiqued, it remains significant to local actors and at the core of prominent political struggles throughout the region.

10. Ibid.

11. Cowen, Dembour, and Wilson 2001, 4–5.

12. Fahmi 2007.

13. "The Islamic Charter for Children vs. Egyptian Law," by Kamilia Helmy (translation by Ashraf Al-Karaksi) published by the International Islamic Committee on Women and Children.

14. Ibid.

15. Fassin 2009: 6–7.

16. Gupta 2012.

17. Ibid., 113.

18. Here, I am drawing on Veena Das (2007), who makes the important claim that we can see politics in small acts and ordinary everyday events, and not only in formal or extraordinary moments.

19. Malkki 2015: 53.

CONCLUSION

1. For more on how responses to the COVID-19 pandemic in the United States speak to the experiences of healthcare workers in the Middle East, see Sweis 2020.

2. Sweis 2017a.

3. Morrison 2015.

4. Fortna 2015.

5. Carpi and Diana 2019.

6. Diana 2019.

7. Ibid., 25.

8. On the limits of street protests in the forging of lasting regime change in Egypt, see especially Bayat 2013a.

9. Nelson 2012.

10. Keraitim and Mehrez 2012: 53–54.

11. Amar 2016: 597.

12. Ticktin 2011: 4.

13. Kleinman and Kleinman 1996.

14. Ibid., 7–8.

15. See "Story of Little Syrian Boy Moves CNN Anchor to Tears," www.cnn.com/videos/world/2016/08/18/syrian-boy-aleppo-omran-bolduan-breaks-down-ath.cnn.

16. Euan McKirdy and Mohammed Tawfeeq, "Omran Daqneesh, Young Face of Aleppo Suffering, Seen on Syrian TV," *CNN World*, June 7, 2017, www.cnn.com/2017/06/07/middleeast/omran-daqneesh-syrian-tv-interview/index.html.

17. Josie Ensor, "'Photo of my dead son has changed nothing,' says father of drowned Syrian refugee boy Alan Kurdi." *The Telegraph* (London), September 3, 2016.

18. Wark 1995: 36.

References

Abramowitz, Sharon, and Catherine Panter-Brick, eds. 2015. *Medical Humanitarianism: Ethnographies of Practice.* Philadelphia: University of Pennsylvania Press.

Abu-Lughod, Lila. 1988. "Fieldwork of a Dutiful Daughter." In *Arab Women in the Field: Studying Your Own Society*, edited by Soraya Altorki and Camillia Fawzi El-Solh, 139–61. Syracuse, NY: Syracuse University Press.

———. 2013. *Do Muslim Women Need Saving?* Cambridge, MA: Harvard University Press.

Ahmed, Leila. 1992. *Women and Gender in Islam.* New Haven, CT: Yale University Press.

Ali, Kamran Asdar. 2002. *Planning the Family in Egypt: New Bodies, New Selves.* Austin: University of Texas Press.

Ali, Nujood, and Delphine Minoui. 2010. *I Am Nujood, Age 10 and Divorced.* New York: Three Rivers Press.

Allen, Lori. 2013. *The Rise and Fall of Human Rights: Cynicism and Politics in Occupied Palestine.* Stanford: Stanford University Press.

Allerton, Catherine. 2018. "Impossible Children: Illegality and Excluded Belonging among Children of Migrants in Sabah, East Malaysia." *Journal of Ethnic and Migration Studies* 44 (7).

Althusser, Louis. 1971. "Ideology and Ideological State Apparatuses (Notes towards an Investigation)." In *The Anthropology of the State: A Reader*, edited by Aradhana Sharma and Akhil Gupta, 86–111. Oxford: Blackwell.

Altorki, Soraya, and Camillia Fawzi El-Solh, eds. 1988. *Arab Women in the Field: Studying Your Own Society*. Syracuse, NY: Syracuse University Press.

Amar, Paul. 2013. *The Security Archipelago: Human-Security States, Sexual Politics, and the End of Neoliberalism*. Durham, NC: Duke University Press.

———. 2016. "The Street, the Sponge, and the Ultra: Queer Logics of Children's Rebellion and Political Infantilization." *GLQ: A Journal of Lesbian and Gay Studies*. doi: 10.1215/10642684-3603102.

Asad, Talal. 2000. "What Do Human Rights Do? An Anthropological Enquiry." *Theory and Event* 4 (4): 1–27.

Bayat, Asef. 2013a. "The Arab Spring and its Surprises." Development and Change. 44 (3): 587–601.

———. 2013b. *Life as Politics: How Ordinary People Change the Middle East*. 2010. 2nd ed. Stanford: Stanford University Press.

Beinin, Joel. 2005. "Political Islam and the New Global Economy." *New Centennial Review* 5 (1): 111–39.

Bhabha, Jacqueline. 2005. "The Child—What Sort of Human?" In *The Humanities in Human Rights: Critique, Language, Politics*, 1526–35. New York: Modern Language Association and Graduate Center, City University of New York.

Biehl, Joao, and Adriana Petryna, eds. 2013. *When People Come First: Critical Studies in Global Health*. Princeton, NJ: Princeton University Press.

Bluebond-Langner, Myra, and Jill E. Korbin. 2008. "Challenges and Opportunities in the Anthropology of Childhoods: An Introduction to 'Children, Childhoods, and Childhood Studies.'" *American Anthropologist* 109 (2): 241–46.

Bornstein, Erica. 2005. *The Spirit of Development: Protestant NGOs, Morality, and Economics in Zimbabwe*. Stanford: Stanford University Press.

Bornstein, Erica and Peter Redfield, ed. 2010. *Forces of Compassion: Humanitarianism between Ethics and Politics*. Santa Fe: School for Advanced Research Press.

Cabot, Heath. 2016. "'Contagious' Solidarity: Reconfiguring Care and Citizenship in Greece's Social Clinics." *Social Anthropology* 24 (2): 152–66.

Caldeira, Teresa P. R. 2000. *City of Walls: Crime, Segregation, and Citizenship in São Paulo*. Berkeley: University of California Press.

Caldron, Paul, Ann Impens, Milena Pavlova, and Wim Groot. 2016. "Economic Assessment of US Physician Participation in Short-term Medical Missions." *Globalization and Health* 12 (45). doi: 10.1186/s12992–016–0183–7.

Carpi, Estella, and Chiara Diana. 2019. "The Right to Play Versus the Right to War? Vulnerable Childhood in Lebanon's NGOization." In *Disadvantaged Childhoods and Humanitarian Intervention*, edited by Kristen Cheney and Aviva Sinervo, 135–56. New York: Palgrave Macmillan.

Chatterjee, Partha. 1989. "Colonialism, Nationalism, and Colonized Women: The Contest in India." *American Ethnologist* 16 (4): 622–33.

Cheney, Kristen E. 2007. *Pillars of the Nation: Child Citizens and Ugandan National Development*. Chicago: University of Chicago Press.

———. 2011. "Children as Ethnographers: Reflections on the Importance of Participatory Research in Assessing Orphans' Needs." *Childhood* 18 (2): 166–79.

Cole, Jennifer, and Deborah Durham. 2007. "Introduction: Age, Regeneration, and the Intimate Politics of Globalization." In *Generations and Globalization: Youth, Age, and Family in the New World Economy*, edited by Jennifer Cole and Deborah Durham, 1–28. Bloomington: Indiana University Press.

Comaroff, Jean, and John L. Comaroff. 2000. "Millennial Capitalism: First Thoughts on a Second Coming." *Public Culture* 12 (2): 291–343.

Cowen, Jane K., Marie-Bénédicte Dembour, and Richard A. Wilson. 2001. "Introduction." In *Culture and Rights: Anthropological Perspectives*, 1–26. Cambridge: Cambridge University Press.

Cox, Aimee Meredith. 2015. *Shapeshifters: Black Girls and the Choreography of Citizenship*. Durham, NC: Duke University Press.

Dahl, Bianca. 2014. "'Too Fat to Be an Orphan': The Moral Semiotics of Food Aid in Botswana." *Cultural Anthropology* 29 (4): 626–47.

———. 2015. "Sexy Orphans and Sugar Daddies: The Sexual and Moral Politics of Aid for AIDS in Botswana." *Studies in Comparative International Development*, September 2015, 1–20.

Das, Veena. 2007. *Life and Words: Violence and the Descent into the Ordinary*. Berkeley: University of California Press.

Diana, Chiara. 2019. "Legitimizing Child Martyrdom? The Emergence of a New Political Subjectivity in Revolutionary Egypt." *Mediterranean Politics*. doi: 10.1080/13629395.2019.1673423.

Dewachi, Omar. 2015. "When Wounds Travel." *Medicine Anthropology Theory* 2 (3): 61–82.

Dumit, Joseph. 2012. *Drugs for Life: How Pharmaceutical Companies Define Our Health*. Durham, NC: Duke University Press.

Dubal, Sam. 2018. *Against Humanity: Lessons from The Lord's Resistance Army*. Oakland: University of California Press.

El-Shewy, Mohamed. 2013. "The Persistence of the Police in Egypt." *Egyptian Initiative for Personal Rights.* August 12.

Elyachar, Julia. 2005. *Markets of Dispossession: NGOs, Economic Development, and the State in Cairo.* Durham, NC: Duke University Press.

Fadlalla, Amal Hassan. 2018. *Branding Humanity: Competing Narratives of Rights, Violence, and Global Citizenship.* Stanford: Stanford University Press.

Fahmi, Kamal. 2007. *Beyond the Victim: The Politics and Ethics of Empowering Cairo's Street Children.* Cairo: American University of Cairo Press.

Fassin, Didier. 2010. "Noli Me Tangere: The Moral Untouchability of Humanitarianism." In *Forces of Compassion: Humanitarianism between Ethics and Politics,* edited by Erica Bornstein and Peter Redfield, 35–52. Santa Fe: School for Advanced Research Press.

———. 2012. *Humanitarian Reason: A Moral History of the Present.* Berkeley: University of California Press.

———. 2013. "Children as Victims: The Moral Economy of Childhood in the Times of AIDS." In *When People Come First: Critical Studies in Global Health,* edited by João Guilherme Biehl and Adriana Petryna, 109–29. Princeton, NJ: Princeton University Press.

Fassin, Didier, and Richard Rechtman. 2009. *The Empire of Trauma: An Inquiry into the Condition of Victimhood.* Princeton, NJ: Princeton University Press.

Feldman, Ilana. 2008. *Governing Gaza: Bureaucracy, Authority, and the Work of Rule, 1917–1967.* Durham, NC: Duke University Press.

Feldman, Ilana, and Miriam Ticktin, eds. 2010. *In the Name of Humanity: The Government of Threat and Care.* Durham, NC: Duke University Press.

Ferguson, James. 1994. *The Anti-Politics Machine: "Development," Depoliticization, and Bureaucratic Power in Lesotho.* Minneapolis: University of Minnesota Press.

———. 2006. *Global Shadows: Africa in the Neoliberal World Order.* Durham, NC: Duke University Press.

Fortna, Benjamin C. 2015. "Preface." In *Childhood in the Late Ottoman Empire and After,* edited by Benjamin C. Fortna, vii–xvii. Brill.

Foucault, Michel. 1977. *Discipline and Punish: the Birth of the Prison.* New York: Vintage Books.

Geertz, Clifford. 1977. *The Interpretation of Cultures.* New York: Basic Books.

Ghannam, Farha. 2013. *Live and Die Like a Man: Gender Dynamics in Urban Egypt.* Stanford: Stanford University Press.

Gordon, Deborah. 1988. "Tenacious Assumptions in Western Biomedicine." In

Biomedicine Examined, edited by Margaret Lock and Deborah Gordon. Dordrecht, Netherlands: Springer.

Gupta, Akhil. 2012. *Red Tape: Bureaucracy, Structural Violence, and Poverty in India.* Durham, NC: Duke University Press.

Hamdy, Sherine F. 2008. "When the State and Your Kidneys Fail: Political Etiologies in an Egyptian Dialysis Ward." *American Ethnologist* 35 (4): 553–69.

———. 2012. *Our Bodies Belong to God: Organ Transplants, Islam, and the Struggle for Human Dignity in Egypt.* Berkeley: University of California Press.

Harvey, David. 2006. *Spaces of Global Capitalism: Towards a Theory of Uneven Geographical Development.* New York: Verso.

Hengeveld, Maria. 2015. "Nike's Girl Effect: The Myth of the Economically Empowered Adolescent Girl." *Al Jazeera America*, July 20. http://america.aljazeera.com/opinions/2015/7/nikes-girl-effect.html.

Henry, Clement M., and Robert Springborg. 2010. *Globalization and the Politics of Development in the Middle East.* New York: Cambridge University Press.

Herrera, Linda, and Asef Bayat, eds. 2010. *Being Young and Muslim: New Cultural Politics in the Global South and North.* Oxford: Oxford University Press.

Honwana, Alcinda, and Filip de Boeck, eds. 2005. *Makers & Breakers: Children & Youth in Postcolonial Africa.* Trenton, NJ: Africa World Press.

Hunleth, Jean. 2013. "Children's Roles in Tuberculosis Treatment Regimes: Constructing Childhood and Kinship in Urban Zambia." *Medical Anthropology Quarterly* 27 (2): 292–311.

Hunleth, Jean, Rebekah Jacob, Steven Cole, Virginia Bond, and Aimee James. 2015. "School Holidays: Examining Childhood, Gender Norms, and Kinship in Children's Shorter-term Residential Mobility in Urban Zambia." *Children's Geographies* 13 (5): 501–17.

Inhorn, Marcia C. 2003. *Local Babies, Global Science: Gender, Religion, and In Vitro Fertilization in Egypt.* New York: Routledge.

James, Erica Caple. 2010. *Democratic Insecurities: Violence, Trauma, and Intervention in Haiti.* Berkeley: University of California Press.

Keraitim, Sahar, and Samia Mehrez. 2012. "Mulid al-Tahrir: Semiotics of a Revolution." In *Translating Egypt's Revolution: The Language of Tahrir*, edited by Sahar Keraitim and Samia Mehrez, 25–67. New York: American University in Cairo Press.

Kleinman, Arthur. 1988. *The Illness Narratives: Suffering, Healing and the Human Condition.* New York: Basic Books.

Kleinman, Arthur, and Joan Kleinman. 1996. "The Appeal of Experience: The Dismay of Images: Cultural Appropriations of Suffering in Our Times." *Dædalus* 125 (1): 1–23.

LeFrancois, Brenda A. 2007. "Children's Participation Rights: Voicing Opinions in Inpatient Care." *Child and Adolescent Mental Health* 12 (2): 94–97.

———. 2013. "The Psychiatrization of Our Children, or, An Autoethnographic Narrative of Perpetuating First Nations Genocide through 'benevolent' Institutions." *Decolonization: Indigeneity, Education & Society* 2 (1): 108–23.

Livingston, Julie. 2012. *Improvising Medicine: An African Oncology Ward in an Emerging Cancer Epidemic*. Durham, NC: Duke University Press.

Lockman, Zachary. 1994. "Imagining the Working Class: Culture, Nationalism, and Class Formation in Egypt, 1899–1914." *Poetics Today* 15 (2): 157–90.

Lotfi, Ali. 2018. "How Premeds Can Maximize International Volunteer Trips." *U.S. News*, August 21. www.usnews.com/education/blogs/medical-school-admissions-doctor/articles/2018-08-21/how-premeds-can-maximize-international-volunteer-trips.

Mahmood, Saba. 2005. *Politics of Piety: the Islamic Revival and the Feminist Subject*. Princeton, NJ: Princeton University Press.

Malkki, Liisa H. 2015. *The Need to Help: The Domestic Arts of International Humanitarianism*. Durham, NC: Duke University Press.

Malkki, Liisa, and Emily Martin. 2003. "Children and the Gendered Politics of Globalization: In Remembrance of Sharon Stephens." *American Ethnologist* 30 (2): 216–24.

Marcus, George E. 1995. "Ethnography in/of the World System: The Emergence of Multi-Sited Ethnography." *Annual Review of Anthropology* 24: 95–117.

Marshall, Andrew Gavin. 2013. "Egypt under Empire, Part 3: From Nasser to Mubarak." *Geopolitics*, July 24.

Marshall, David Jones. 2014. "Save (us from) the Children: Trauma, Palestinian Childhood, and the Production of Governable Subjects." *Children's Geographies* 12 (1): 281–96. doi: 10.1080/14733285.2014.922678.

Martin, Emily. 2007. *Bipolar Expeditions: Mania and Depression in American Culture*. Princeton, NJ: Princeton University Press.

Mattingly, Cheryl. 2010. *The Paradox of Hope: Journeys through a Clinical Borderland*. Berkeley: University of California Press.

Mauss, Marcel. 2000 [1925]. *The Gift: The Form and Reason for Exchange in Archaic Societies*. New York: Norton.

McKay, Ramah 2012. "Afterlives: Humanitarian Histories and Critical Subjects in Mozambique." *Cultural Anthropology* 27 (2): 286–309.

———. 2018. *Medicine in the Meantime: The Work of Care in Mozambique.* Durham, NC: Duke University Press.

Merry, Sally Engle. 2006. *Human Rights & Gender Violence: Translating International Law into Local Justice.* Chicago: University of Chicago Press.

Metzl, Jonathan M. 2009. *The Protest Psychosis: How Schizophrenia Became a Black Disease.* Boston: Beacon Press.

Mitchell, Timothy. 2002. *Rule of Experts: Egypt, Techno-Politics, Modernity.* Berkeley: University of California Press.

Mohanty, Chandra Talpade. 1988. "Under Western Eyes: Feminist Scholarship and Colonial Discourses." *Feminist Review* 30 (Autumn): 61–88.

Montgomery, Heather. 2001. "Imposing Rights? A Case Study of Child Prostitution in Thailand." In *Culture and Rights: Anthropological Perspectives,* edited by Jane K. Cowan, Marie-Bénédicte Dembour, and Richard A. Wilson, 80–101. Cambridge: Cambridge University Press.

———. 2009. *An Introduction to Childhood: Anthropological Perspectives on Children's Lives.* Oxford: Wiley-Blackwell.

Morrison, Heidi. 2015. *Childhood and Colonial Modernity in Egypt.* New York, NY: Palgrave Macmillan.

Negrón-Gonzales, Geneviève. 2016. "Teaching Poverty." In Ananya Roy, Geneviève Negrón-Gonzales, Kweku Opoku-Agyemang, and Clare Vineeta Talwalker, *Encountering Poverty: Thinking and Acting in an Unequal World,* 149–78. Oakland: University of California Press.

Nelson, Soraya Sarhaddi. 2012. "Egypt's Street Kids Are Revolution's Smallest Soldiers." NPR. www.npr.org/2012/01/04/144692425/egypts-street-kids-are-revolutions-smallest-soldiers.

Nguyen, Vinh-Kim. 2010. *The Republic of Therapy: Triage and Sovereignty in West Africa's Time of AIDS.* Durham, NC: Duke University Press.

Okuma, Teruo. 1983. "Therapeutic and Prophylactic Effects of Carbamazepine in Bipolar Disorders." *Psychiatric Clinic of North America* 6 (1): 157–74.

Omidian, Patricia, and Catherine Panter-Brick. 2015. "Dignity under Extreme Duress: The Moral and Emotional Landscape of Local Humanitarian Workers in the Afghan-Pakistan Border Areas." In *Medical Humanitarianism: Ethnographies of Practice,* edited by Sharon Abramowitz and Catherine Panter-Brick, 23–40. Philadelphia: University of Pennsylvania Press.

O'Neill, Bruce. 2014. "Cast Aside: Boredom, Downward Mobility, and Homelessness in Post-Communist Bucharest." *Cultural Anthropology* 29 (1): 8–31.

Ong, Aihwa. 2006. *Neoliberalism as Exception: Mutations in Citizenship and Sovereignty*. Durham, NC: Duke University Press.

Orellana, Marjorie Faulstich. 2009. *Translating Childhoods: Immigrant Youth, Language, and Culture*. New Brunswick, NJ: Rutgers University Press.

Redfield, Peter. 2013. *Life in Crisis: The Ethical Journey of Doctors Without Borders*. Berkeley: University of California Press.

Rose, Nikolas. 2006. *The Politics of Life Itself: Biomedicine, Power, and Subjectivity in the Twenty-First Century*. Princeton, NJ: Princeton University Press.

Roy, Ananya. 2010. *Poverty Capital: Microfinance and the Making of Development*. New York: Routledge.

Roy, Ananya, Geneviève Negrón-Gonzales, Kweku Opoku-Agyemang, and Clare Vineeta Talwalker. *Encountering Poverty: Thinking and Acting in an Unequal World*. Oakland: University of California Press.

Said, Edward. 1979. *Orientalism*. New York: Vintage Books.

Samaan, Magdy. 2008. "Shoura Council Passes Child Law, Criminalizes FGM." *Daily News Egypt*, May 12.

Sanford III, Ezelle, and Chelsey Carter. 2020. "From Spanish Flu to COVID-19: Race, Class and Reopening St. Louis." *Riverfront Times*, May 13. www.riverfronttimes.com/stlouis/from-spanish-flu-to-covid-19-race-class-and-reopening-st-louis/Content?oid=33546386.

Sassen, Saskia. 2001. *The Global City: New York, London, Tokyo*. 2nd ed. Princeton, NJ: Princeton University Press.

Scheper-Hughes, Nancy, and Carolyn Sargent. 1998. "Introduction: the Cultural Politics of Childhood." In *Small Wars: The Cultural Politics of Childhood*, edited by Nancy. Scheper-Hughes and Carolyn Sargent, 1–33. Berkeley: University of California Press.

Scheper-Hughes, Nancy, and Daniel Hoffman. 1998. "Brazilian Apartheid: Street Kids and the Struggle for Urban Space." In *Small Wars: The Cultural Politics of Childhood*, edited by Nancy Scheper-Hughes and Carolyn Sargent, 352–88. Berkeley: University of California Press.

Schwartzman, Helen B. 2011 [1978]. *Transformations: The Anthropology of Children's Play*. eBook. Boston: Springer US. www.springer.com/gp/book/9781461339403.

Shepler, Susan. 2005. "The Rites of the Child: Global Discourses of Youth and Reintegrating Child Soldiers in Sierra Leone." *Journal of Human Rights* 4: 197–211.

Simone, Abdou Maliq. 2004. *For the City Yet to Come: Changing African Life in Four Cities.* Durham, NC: Duke University Press.

Sinervo, Aviva. 2013. "'No somos los pobrecitos': Negotiating Stigma, Identity, and Need in Constructions of Childhood Poverty in Cusco, Peru." *Childhood* 20 (3): 1–16.

Sinervo, Aviva, and Michael D. Hill. 2011. "The Visual Economy of Andean Childhood Poverty: Interpreting Postcards in Cusco, Peru." *Journal of Latin American and Caribbean Anthropology* 16 (1): 114–42.

Singerman, Diane, and Paul Amar, eds. 2006. *Cairo Cosmopolitan: Politics, Culture, and Urban Space in the New Globalized Middle East.* New York: American University in Cairo Press.

Stephens, Sharon ed. 1995. *Children and the Politics of Culture.* Princeton, NJ: Princeton University Press.

Sweis, Rania Kassab. 2012. "Saving Egypt's Village Girls: Humanity, Rights, and Gendered Vulnerability in a Global Youth Initiative." *Journal of Middle East Women's Studies* 8 (2): 26–50.

———. 2017a. "Children as Biological Sufferers? The Paradox of International Medical Aid for Homeless Children in Cairo." *Childhood* 24 (4): 502–16.

———. 2017b. "Do Muslim Village Girls Need Saving? Critical Reflections on Gender and Childhood Suffering in International Aid." In *The Global Status of Women and Girls: A Multidisciplinary Approach*, edited by Lori Underwood and Dawn Hutchinson, 105–14. Lanham, MD: Lexington Books.

———. 2017c. "Security and the Traumatized Street Child: How Gender Shapes International Psychiatric Aid in Cairo." *Medical Anthropology Quarterly* 32 (1): 5–21.

———. 2020. "Hospital Warzones: What Syrian and U.S. Health Workers Now Share." *Globe Post*, April 22.

Ticktin, Miriam. 2006. "Where Ethics and Politics Meet: The Violence of Humanitarianism in France." *American Ethnologist* 33 (1): 33–49.

———. 2011. *Casualties of Care: Immigration and the Politics of Humanitarianism in France.* Berkeley: University of California Press.

Tsing, Anna Lowenhaupt. 2005. *Friction: An Ethnography of Global Connection.* Princeton, NJ: Princeton University Press.

Vaughan, Megan. 1991. *Curing Their Ills: Colonial Power and African Illness.* Stanford: Stanford University Press.

Wark, McKenzie. 1995. "Fresh Maimed Babies: The Uses of Innocence." *Transition* (65): 36–47.

Wendland, Claire L. 2010. *A Heart for the Work: Journeys through an African Medical System*. Chicago: University of Chicago Press.

Winegar, Jessica. 2006. *Creative Reckonings: The Politics of Art and Culture in Contemporary Egypt*. Stanford: Stanford University Press.

Winegar, Jessica, and Amahl Bishara. 2009. "Culture Concepts in Political Struggle." *Review of Middle East Studies* 43 (2): 164–67.

Index

Abu-Lughod, Lila: on emancipation and Egyptian women, 97–98; on gendered orientalism, 97–98
Afghanistan, 161
Africa, 9, 11; aid for children in, 110, 112, 122, 162, 166n22; biomedicine in, 166n21; child soldiers in, 32; neoliberalism in, 13; sub-Saharan Africa, 9, 13, 122. *See also* North Africa
aid workers: attitudes of, 5, 6–7, 9–10, 14–15, 19–20, 21, 93, 99, 100, 109–10, 111–12, 113, 114–16, 123, 124–29, 130, 132–34, 135–49, 152, 154–55, 158–59, 162, 163, 171n3; attitudes regarding detention of children, 125–26, 129, 132, 133, 136–40, 143, 144; attitudes regarding Egypt's culture and children's rights, 133, 135–36, 139–46; attitudes regarding Egypt's national development, 114–16, 123; attitudes regarding fund-raising, 93, 99, 100, 111–12, 113, 116, 147; attitudes regarding social justice, 109, 111–12, 133, 135, 138, 140, 141, 148, 149; attitudes regarding villages, 105, 107–8, 109–10, 114–16; as cultural intermediaries, 128, 133, 140, 146, 148, 154–55; double consciousness among, 128, 132–34; foreign-born professionals vs. local aid workers, 58; as global citizens, 127–28, 171n3; harmful effects on, 3; and healthy childhood discourse, 9, 21–27; humanitarian doctors, 42–46, 47, 50, 57, 58–61, 62–63, 65, 66, 67, 68, 71–74, 75, 82–87, 90, 154–55, 163; improvisation by, 10, 62, 68, 152, 154, 166n21; negotiation by, 10, 46, 58, 62, 69, 82–87, 111, 113, 123, 128, 133, 135, 140, 148; relations with children, 2–3, 7, 8–9, 10–11, 19–21, 26, 27, 28, 33–35, 36, 39, 40, 42–46, 47, 50–51, 52–53, 54–55, 56–58, 60, 62–66, 68, 71–74, 75, 76–80, 81, 88, 90, 91, 92, 96, 101–2, 138–39, 151, 153–54, 168n10; relations with state authorities, 3, 10, 124–27, 128–29, 130,

185

133, 136–40, 142, 144–46, 148, 152, 153, 154–55; religion among, 139; sense of ambivalence among, 111–12, 127–29, 132–34, 147–48, 154, 162
Allen, Lori: on human rights activists in Palestine, 132–33; *The Rise and Fall of Human Rights*, 132–33
Althusser, Louis: on hailing, 168n10, 170n8
antidepressants, 85, 86, 90, 170n17
Arab Spring, 157–59
attitudes regarding children: as autonomous subjects, 7, 30, 39–40, 53, 131, 151, 160; as dependent on adults, 4, 7, 29, 39–40, 47, 48, 51, 55, 68, 79, 80, 88, 151, 157, 160; as emotionally traumatized, 27, 36, 47, 52, 53, 55, 70–74, 75–76, 78, 82, 83, 84, 88, 91, 162; as the future, 110–11; as innocent, 7, 10, 76, 80, 81, 93, 95, 100, 103, 115, 121, 122, 162, 166n22; as martyrs, 157–58, 159; as passive/submissive, 4, 7, 8, 9, 28, 32, 35, 39–40, 48, 51, 54, 55, 68, 76, 78, 79, 80, 97, 151, 154, 155, 156, 157, 160; as political subjects, 155, 157–59; as potential threats, 10, 71, 73, 74, 75, 76–77, 79, 81, 82–83, 85, 92, 123, 143, 153, 156, 169n2; as undeveloped subjects, 55, 160

Beni Suef, 94, 95, 97, 107–8, 115, 116–18
biomedicine, 23, 25, 156, 161; improvisation in, 10, 62, 68, 152, 154, 166n21; and international children's rights, 21, 31, 47, 53, 148, 153, 154; and poor women, 66–67, 168n22; rejected by children, 8, 40, 63–64, 68, 84, 85, 86, 87, 90–91, 154, 160. *See also* medications
Bishara, Amahl, 171n9
Bornstein, Erica: on medical humanitarianism, 4

Brazil: street children in, 91

Cairo, 22, 43, 44, 50, 79, 86, 167n1
Camp David Accords, 12
Carter, Chelsey, 165n9
CCI. *See* Children's Charity International
Chatterjee, Partha, 95, 116
Cheney, Kristen: on children and ethnographic research, 166n12
childhood: as distinct life-phase, 28, 29–30, 157; healthy childhood discourse, 9, 21–27; international model of, 50, 51; Western model of, 28, 29–30, 31–32
Child Law in Egypt, 28–31, 65, 129, 141–46; Article 3, 30–31; Article 31-bis, 29–30; Article 112, 29; and child abuse, 30–31, 131, 134, 135–36, 137, 139–40, 142–43, 144, 145, 153; and marriage age, 29–30, 31, 134; as paradoxical, 30, 31
children: agency of, 1, 7–8, 15, 20–22, 30–31, 32, 35–39, 40–41, 43–44, 45–46, 47–48, 62, 63–64, 73, 78–79, 84, 87, 88–89, 90–91, 110, 122, 151–52, 154, 155, 156, 157–59, 160, 161, 166n12; during Arab Spring, 157–59; attitudes of, 5, 7, 14, 43–44, 45–46, 72–73, 74, 87–92, 97, 117–19, 154, 155; child abuse, 30–31, 131, 134, 135–36, 137, 139–40, 142–43, 144, 145, 153; depiction of, 152, 161–63; detention of, 29, 65, 66, 68, 125–26, 129, 132, 133, 136–40, 143, 144; discipline of, 9, 19, 20, 21, 35, 40–41, 153, 154, 156; Egypt's Child Law, 28–31, 65, 129, 131; in global aid policy, 7, 8, 9, 11–12, 13–14, 26–28, 35, 40, 47, 48, 68, 70, 75–76, 90, 93–94, 97, 99–101, 110–11, 113–14, 127–28, 129, 151, 152, 153, 154, 156, 157, 160, 162; global aid policy regarding, 7, 8, 9, 13–14, 26–27; as independent, 8, 21, 28, 35, 40, 47, 73, 78–79, 87, 89, 90–91; medical

INDEX 187

noncompliance among, 8, 40, 63–64, 68, 84, 85, 86, 87, 90–91, 154, 160; negotiation by, 20, 32, 69, 87, 91, 110, 152, 154, 156, 160, 164; pain experienced by, 47, 52–55, 63–64, 66, 68, 81; as powerful, 20, 21, 40, 110, 166n12; relations with aid workers, 2–3, 7, 8–9, 10–11, 19–21, 26, 27, 28, 33–35, 36, 39, 40, 42–46, 47, 50–51, 52–53, 54–55, 56–58, 60, 62–66, 68, 71–74, 75, 76–80, 81, 88, 90, 91, 92, 96, 101–2, 151, 153–54, 168n10; relations with other children, 21, 87, 88; relations with parents, 102, 108, 109, 131, 135, 139–40, 142–43, 145, 166n22; relations with police, 1, 8, 10, 29, 36, 56, 62, 65–66, 68, 69, 76, 85, 87, 89, 125–26, 127, 129, 130, 131, 132, 137–40, 143, 144, 154, 156; rights of, 7, 14, 15, 17, 21, 27–32, 28, 29, 31, 39–41, 48, 50, 51, 53, 62, 90, 100, 101, 103–5, 108, 114, 118, 120, 126, 127, 131, 133, 134, 135–36, 137, 139–46, 147, 155; self-care among, 47–48; suffering of, 1–2, 3, 7, 8, 9, 62, 66, 69, 70, 74–76, 80, 83, 84, 93, 94, 97, 99, 100, 110, 121, 122, 151, 153, 155, 156, 159, 160, 161–64; universal conceptualizations of, 9, 23, 28, 32, 47, 70–71, 95, 99, 101, 102, 110, 122, 151, 153, 154, 156, 160; as victims, 6, 8, 9, 76, 81, 93, 94, 100, 103, 110, 113–14, 115, 120, 121, 122, 136, 151, 153, 155; as vulnerable, 6, 7, 8, 10, 11, 12, 14, 15, 17, 20, 21, 26, 27, 29, 31, 36, 47, 54, 57–58, 73–74, 78, 79, 80, 81, 92, 99, 101, 103, 107, 122, 129–30, 131, 136, 143, 144, 148, 149, 154, 155, 156, 157, 158, 160, 161. *See also* attitudes regarding children; childhood; Child Law in Egypt; gender

Children's Charity International (CCI): and children's rights, 17, 21, 27–32, 50, 51, 62; and Egypt's Child Law, 28–30; foreign-born professionals vs. local aid workers, 58; form for psychiatric examinations, 82–83; fund-raising by, 49, 74, 78; and GAC, 126, 134; and IVGP, 100; medical-social approach of, 52–55, 62; mission statement, 74; Paris headquarters, 17, 23, 52, 77, 78; policy regarding street children, 19, 21, 23, 27, 40, 51, 52, 62, 64, 66, 67, 71, 74, 79–80, 81, 87, 88–89; psychiatric program, 70–92. *See also* children's shelter of CCI; mobile medical clinic of CCI

children's shelter of CCI, 17–41, 42, 153, 158; admission to, 76–80, 81; children who leave and return to, 36–37, 79, 80, 86, 90–91; compassion at, 21, 35, 36, 40, 45, 47, 54, 70, 71, 76, 77, 79, 81, 91; director of, 77–80, 81, 125; discipline and regulation at, 19, 20, 21, 35, 40–41, 76, 78; education at, 25–26, 27; files kept on children at, 77–78; food at, 23–24; humanitarian doctors at, 71–74, 75, 82–87, 90; hygiene practices at, 21, 24–25, 27, 33–35, 39, 51; innovation at, 17; lice treatments at, 33–35, 40; location, 18, 19, 22; mandatory care at, 27–28, 33–35, 72–73, 75, 86, 90, 91; psychiatric interventions at, 70–76, 82–87, 90, 91; security guard at, 80–81. *See also* mobile medical clinic of CCI

class, 55–56, 57, 66, 168n22

Clinton, Hillary, 95

Cole, Jennifer: on globalization and children, 166n18

colonialism, 5–6, 97, 98, 111

community pharmacies, 43–44, 46, 167n1

compassion, 159, 160, 162–63; vs. discipline, 153, 154; for village girls, 93–94, 95–96, 100, 101

coronavirus pandemic, 2, 3, 4, 5, 152, 161

188   INDEX

cultural intermediaries, 128, 133, 140, 146, 148, 154–55
cultural stereotypes, 12, 96, 98, 110, 111, 160, 164, 166n22

Daqneesh, Omran: image of, 152, 162–63
Das, Veena: on politics in small acts, 172n18
de Boeck, Filip: on child soldiers, 168n17
detention of children, 65, 66, 68; attitudes of aid workers regarding, 125–26, 129, 132, 133, 136–40, 143, 144; in Egypt's Child Law, 29, 136
Diana, Chiara: on street children during Arab Spring, 157, 158
Doctors Without Borders, 5, 48, 53
donors: ExxonMobil, 12, 101, 130, 156; Ford Foundation, 101, 130; Johnson & Johnson, 130; Nike, 12, 101, 156. *See also* fund-raising
drug use, 54, 84
Durham, Deborah: on globalization and children, 166n18

Egypt: Child Law, 28–31, 65, 129, 131, 134–36, 137, 139–40, 141–46; class in, 55–56, 57, 66, 168n22; culture in, 133, 135–36, 139–46, 171n9; divorce in, 78; economic conditions, 11, 12–13, 48, 58, 97–98, 122, 154, 156; global aid policy regarding, 11–14, 151; government policies, 6, 22, 28–30, 65, 86, 97–98, 102, 122, 124–27, 128–29, 142, 147, 167n2; homelessness in, 78; marriage age in, 29–30, 31, 134; mobile medicine vs. public healthcare in, 44, 48–49, 68, 69; National Council of Childhood and Motherhood (NCCM), 29; neoliberalism in, 12–13; political conditions, 86, 155, 157–59; poverty in, 6, 8, 11–12, 13, 55–56, 66–67, 86, 88, 90, 93, 94, 95, 96, 98, 100, 102, 115, 116, 117, 153, 155, 158, 167n2; public education in, 88–89, 117; public healthcare in, 7, 44, 45, 48, 66, 68, 167n1; relations with Israel, 12; relations with United States, 6, 11, 12; rural vs. urban, 102, 103, 108, 114–16, 123; state authority vs. parental authority in, 131, 135, 139–40, 142–43, 145; tourism in, 22, 23, 27, 35–39; unemployment in, 11; U.S. foreign aid to, 6, 11; young population in, 11–13
el-Sisi, Abdel Fattah, 159
ethnographic research, 14–15, 48, 60, 62, 96, 97, 145, 168n22, 169n23; and globalization, 166n14; as multi-site, 7, 166n12; participant-observation in, 24; qualitative approaches in, 3, 151
European Commission, 130
ExxonMobil, 12, 101, 130, 156

Fadlalla, Amal Hassan: on global citizenship, 171n3
Fassin, Didier: on hierarchies of suffering, 166n22; on humanitarianism, 10, 71–72, 144, 166n22; on humanitarian psychiatry, 71–72
Feldman, Ilana: on providers vs. recipients of aid, 58
feminism, 114, 123; transnational feminist scholars, 98
Ferguson, James: on state-NGO relations, 130–31
Ford Foundation, 101, 130
Foucault, Michel, 9
France, 5, 6; colonialism of, 11, 111; Muslim immigrants in, 109
fund-raising, 1–2, 3–4, 13, 49, 78, 163; attitudes of aid workers regarding, 93,

99, 100, 111–12, 113, 116, 147; by CCI, 49, 74, 78; by GAC, 130; major donors, 12, 101, 130, 156; role of images of children in, 74, 100; by USDI/IVGP, 93, 97, 99, 100, 101, 111–12, 113, 116, 121, 122

GAC. *See* Global Aid for Children
Gaza, 11, 17, 48, 161
gender: boys as potential threats, 10, 71, 73, 74, 75, 76–77, 79, 81, 82–83, 85, 92, 123, 143, 153, 156, 169n2; exposure of village girls to males, 107, 108–9; feminized characteristics and aid workers, 136–37; gendered hierarchy of care, 10, 71, 73–74, 75, 76, 80–82, 153; gendered orientalism, 97–98; gendered violence, 93, 96, 99, 103, 114, 123, 153; girls' attitudes regarding marriage, 118, 119–20, 121; girls vs. boys, 10, 26, 49–50, 73–74, 75, 76, 78–79, 80–81, 85, 104–5, 108–9, 123, 153, 156; normative models of masculinity, 88, 90, 91, 169n13; patriarchal authority, 94, 95, 100, 140; psychiatric intervention for boys, 71, 73–74, 75, 76; puberty for girls, 99–100; self-inflicted wounds among males, 65, 66; shared masculine precarity, 56–58; smoking among street boys, 50–51, 61, 63, 66
Ghannam, Farha: on masculinity in Cairo, 79, 169n13
Girl Up program, 3–4, 95–96, 170n8
Giza, 56, 70; Pyramids, 22–23, 35–36, 38–39, 88, 89
Global Aid for Children (GAC), 133–36, 158, 171n3; and Egypt's Child Law, 134–36, 137, 139–40, 141–46; funding for, 130; relations with state authorities, 124–27, 128–32, 146–47, 148

global aid policy: children in, 7, 8, 9, 11–12, 13–14, 26–28, 35, 40, 47, 48, 68, 70, 75–76, 90, 93–94, 97, 99–101, 110–11, 113–14, 127–28, 129, 151, 152, 153, 154, 156, 157, 160, 162; Egypt in, 11–12, 151; gender in, 75–76; health and children's rights in, 27–28, 90; vs. local implementation, 10, 14, 86, 110; role of cultural stereotypes in, 12, 98, 110, 111, 153, 160, 164; and social justice, 160–61; street children in, 26–27, 70, 75–76, 152, 154; village girls in, 93–94, 97, 99–101, 113–14, 152, 153, 154
global citizenship, 127–28, 171n3
global health industry, 4, 6–7, 156, 161–62, 163
global inequality, 14
globalization, 13, 166n14
global north: cultural stereotypes in, 12, 96, 98, 110, 111, 160, 164, 166n22; domination of global south, 4; vs. global south, 32; medical missions from, 5
global studies students, 2, 4
Gordon, Deborah: on human rights and biomedicine, 53; "Tenacious Assumptions in Western Biomedicine", 53
Gupta, Akhil: on state narratives, 145–46

hailing, 51, 168n10, 170n8
Hamdy, Sherine: on ethics and Egyptian healthcare, 167n2
healthy childhood discourse, 9, 21–27
Hecht, Tobias: on street children in Brazil, 91
Honwana, Alcinda: on child soldiers, 168n17
humanitarian aid: as beneficial, 5, 7, 9, 10, 153–54; as harmful/limiting, 2, 3, 5, 7, 8, 9, 87, 154; humanitarian crises

in Middle East and North Africa, 11; medical aid outcomes, 7, 9, 40, 42, 46, 63, 79, 151, 153, 154–55; as paradoxical, 2–3, 7, 9–10, 14, 15, 21, 40–41, 45, 46, 69, 71, 96, 120–21, 127, 153–54, 160; vs. structural conditions, 2–3, 5, 7, 9, 39, 40, 45, 69, 86, 96, 120–21, 154, 160, 161, 161–62, 163–64; unintended consequences of, 4, 10, 62, 120–21. *See also* global aid policy

humanitarian government and hierarchy, 9

Hunleth, Jean, 8, 60

hygiene practices, 21, 24–25, 27, 33–35, 39, 51

I am Nujood, Age 10 and Divorced, 94–96, 97, 98

illness narratives, 47–48, 62, 68

India, 145

Inhorn, Marcia C.: on women and biomedicine, 168n22

international aid organizations, 13, 26, 117; relations with the state, 124–27, 128–32, 146–47, 148, 158–59. *See also* Children's Charity International (CCI); Global Aid for Children (GAC); International Village Girl Project (IVGP); United States Development Initiative (USDI)

international children's rights: and biomedicine, 21, 31, 47, 53, 148, 153, 154; local implementation, 14, 62, 127–29, 131–32, 133–36, 137, 139–40, 142–44, 148–49; model of the child in, 7, 15, 28, 31–32, 39–40, 48, 50, 51, 95, 131, 151, 156, 157, 164; relationship to children's health, 27–32

International Committee of the Red Cross (ICRC), 48

International Monetary Fund, 6, 13

International Village Girl Project (IVGP): attitudes of aid workers at, 93–94, 96–97, 99, 105–16, 121–22, 123; attitudes of aid workers regarding fund-raising, 111–12, 113, 116; attitudes of aid workers regarding national development, 114–16, 123; attitudes of aid workers regarding successes of, 113–14; attitudes of aid workers regarding villages, 105, 107–8, 109–10, 114–16; attitudes of village girls regarding, 117–21; and children's rights, 101, 103–5, 108, 114, 118, 120; demographer at, 114–15; director of, 93–94, 99, 109–10, 111–12, 113, 116, 122, 123; and domestic labor, 118, 120–21; dress (*libs*) promoted by, 103, 118; exercise (*harakat al-gism*) promoted by, 103, 104; expansion of, 122; fund-raising for, 93, 97, 99, 100, 101, 111–12, 113, 116, 121, 122; global youth habitus promoted by, 102, 103, 118; goals of, 101, 102–3; hygienic practices (*nadafa*) promoted by, 103, 118; and indoors-outdoors distinction, 104; and marriage, 118, 120, 121; and morality, 103–4, 107, 111–12, 114; multilingualism among aid workers, 106, 112–13; origin, 100–101; othering discourses at, 96, 114–15, 122, 123; project manager of, 112–13; and right to play, 103–5; and USDI, 100–101, 106–7, 113–15, 123

Iraq, 11, 48, 161

Islam, 96, 98, 111, 122, 153; Islamic extremism, 11, 95, 110, 114–15, 122–23, 142; Sharia (Islamic law), 30

Islamophobia, 110

IVGP. *See* International Village Girl Project

Johns Hopkins University's COVID-19 Dashboard, 2

Johnson & Johnson, 130

Kleinman, Arthur: on illness narratives, 47–48, 62
Kleinman, Arthur and Joan: on appropriation of suffering, 161–62
Kurdi, Alan, 163

Latin America: neoliberalism in, 13
Lebanon, 17, 48
lice treatment, 33–35, 40
Livingston, Julie: on improvisation in biomedicine, 166n21

Malinowski, Bronislaw, 24
Malkki, Liisa: on attitudes of aid workers, 147; on children as good investments, 110; on tranquilizing conventions, 100
Marcus, George: on globalization and ethnographic research, 166n14
marriage, 58, 99, 131; child marriage in Yemen, 94, 95, 98, 100; girls' attitudes regarding, 97, 118, 119–20, 121; legal age in Egypt, 29–30, 31, 134; *urfi* marriage, 30
Marshall, David: on Palestinian children, 169n2
Mattingly, Cheryl: on medical charts, 83
McKay, Ramah, 10
Mead Margaret, 24
Médecins du Monde (MDM), 53
Médecins Sans Frontières (MSF), 5, 48, 53
medical humanitarianism: vs. economic/political processes, 4–5; as industry, 4; medical aid outcomes, 7, 9, 40, 42, 46, 63, 79, 151, 153, 154–55; as medical missions, 5–6
medical missions, 5–6
medical students, 4

medications, 4, 5, 21, 25, 63–64; lice treatments, 33–35, 40; psychotropic medications, 71, 73, 77, 82, 84–86, 87, 90, 91–92, 170n17; Tegretol, 85, 86, 90, 170n17. *See also* biomedicine
mental health. *See* psychiatric care
Merry, Sally Engle: on vernacularization, 128, 133
Metzl, Jonathan: on racialization of schizophrenia, 75
Middle East: colonization in, 11, 97; culture concept in, 171n9; global aid policy regarding, 11–12, 142, 160, 161, 164; humanitarian crisis in, 11; and international children's rights, 28; mobile medicine in, 48–49; neoliberalism in, 13; nongovernmental organizations in, 13, 28; refugees from, 161; village girls in, 93–94, 97
Middle East Studies, 6
Minoui, Delphine, 94–95
Mitchell, Timothy, 115
mobile medical clinic of CCI, 41, 153; care provided by, 42–47, 49–50, 51, 60–62, 63–67, 68, 69; vs. CCI shelter, 46, 50; vs. community pharmacy, 43–44, 46; education at, 50–51, 168n10; gift bags distributed by, 49–50, 51, 66, 168n10; hailing by aid workers, 51, 168n10; homeless boys as patients, 42–46, 47, 156, 158; local aid workers of, 58; paradoxes of assistance by, 45, 46; pedagogical lectures at, 50–51; relations with poor urban women, 66–67
Mohanty, Chandra: on Muslim village girls and aid policy, 100
Montgomery, Heather: on child prostitution in Thailand, 32
Morocco, 17

Morsi, Mohamed, 159
Mozambique, 10
Mubarak, Hosni, 158, 159
multilingualism, 106, 112–13, 148
Muslim Brotherhood, 30, 158–59

negotiation: by aid workers, 10, 46, 58, 62, 69, 82–87, 111, 113, 123, 128, 133, 135, 140, 148; by children, 20, 32, 69, 87, 91, 110, 152, 154, 156, 160, 164
neoliberalism, 12–13, 28, 69, 98, 153
Nike, 12, 101, 156
Nile River, 11
North Africa: humanitarian crisis in, 11; Muslim village girls in, 93–94, 97; nongovernmental organizations in, 13

Okuma, Teruo, 170n17
O'Neill, Bruce, 169n23
online donation funds, 3

Palestine: Gaza, 11, 17, 48, 161; human rights activists in, 132–33; traumatized children in, 169n2
paradoxes: regarding aid workers, 2–3, 147, 152, 153, 154; regarding Child Law in Egypt, 30, 31; regarding conceptions of children, 92, 110; definition of paradox, 2; regarding humanitarian aid, 2–3, 7, 9–10, 14, 15, 21, 40–41, 45, 46, 69, 71, 96, 120–21, 127, 153–54, 160; regarding international children's rights, 127–29; as requiring qualitative approaches in research methods, 3
patriarchy, 94, 95, 100, 140
police: detention of children by, 29, 65, 66, 68, 125–26, 129, 132, 133, 136–40, 143; militarization of, 13; relations with street children, 1, 8, 10, 29, 36, 56, 62, 65–66, 68, 69, 76, 85, 87, 89, 125–26, 127, 129, 130, 131, 132, 137–40, 143, 144, 154, 156
population control, 102
psychiatric care, 70–92, 153; antidepressants in, 85, 86, 90, 170n17; psychiatric intervention for boys, 71, 73–74, 75, 76

Rechtman, Richard: on humanitarian psychiatry, 71–72
Redfield, Peter: on medical humanitarianism, 4; on mobile medicine, 48, 69
religious conservatism, 93, 95, 97, 101, 110, 114–15, 134, 153
Roy, Ananya, 11
rural villages vs. cities, 102, 103, 108, 114–16, 123

Sadat, Anwar: economic policies, 12
Said, Edward: *Orientalism*, 97
Sanford III, Ezelle, 165n9
September 11th attacks, 11–12
Sharia (Islamic law), 30
Shubra al Khaima, 57, 61, 63
smoking, 50–51, 61, 63, 66, 84, 91
social justice, 8, 15, 158, 160–61, 164; attitudes of aid workers regarding, 109, 111–12, 133, 135, 138, 140, 141, 148, 149. *See also* structural conditions
South Africa: HIV/AIDS in, 166n22
Spanish Flu pandemic, 165n9
state authorities: vs. parental authority, 131, 135, 139–40, 142–43, 145; relations with aid workers, 3, 10, 124–27, 128–29, 130, 133, 136–40, 142, 144–46, 148, 152, 153, 154–55; relations with international aid organizations, 124–27, 128–32, 146–47, 148, 158–59

street children, 7, 10, 13–14, 152; in Article 112 of Child Law, 29, 31; in CCI policy, 19, 21, 23, 27, 40, 51, 52, 62, 64, 66, 67, 70, 71, 73, 74, 79–80, 81, 87, 88–89; as crisis in Egypt, 23, 59, 86, 126; defined, 19, 29, 31; foot wounds among, 45, 61; relations with police, 1, 8, 10, 29, 36, 56, 62, 65–66, 68, 69, 76, 85, 87, 89, 125–26, 127, 129, 130, 131, 132, 137–40, 143, 144, 154, 156; stomach infections among, 61; working near Pyramids, 22–23, 35–36, 38–39, 88, 89. *See also* Children's Charity International (CCI); children's shelter of CCI; Global Aid for Children (GAC); mobile medical clinic of CCI; psychiatric care

structural conditions, 12–13, 32, 54, 110, 115, 116, 152, 155; vs. humanitarian aid, 2–3, 5, 7, 9, 39, 40, 45, 69, 86, 96, 120–21, 154, 160, 161, 161–62, 163–64; poverty and violence as, 5, 8, 32, 39, 41, 156

sub-Saharan Africa: neoliberalism in, 13

Syria, 11, 48, 161; image of Alan Kurdi, 163; image of Omran Daqneesh, 152, 162–63

Tegretol, 85, 86, 90, 170n17
television aid advertisements, 1–2
Thailand: child prostitution in, 32
Ticktin, Miriam: on medical missions, 5
tourism, 22, 23, 27, 35–39
Tsing, Anna: on frictions in global aid, 127

United Kingdom, 6, 11
United Nations, 130, 142; Girl Up program, 3–4, 95–96, 170n8
United Nations Children's Fund (UNICEF), on humanitarian crises in Middle East and North Africa, 11
United Nations Convention on the Rights of the Child (UNCRC), 28, 29, 31, 127, 131, 134
United Nations High Commissioner for Refugees (UNHCR), 58; on humanitarian crises in Middle East and North Africa, 11
United Nations Relief and Works Agency for Palestinian Refugees (UNRWA), 58
United States: African Americans, 5, 165n9; angry black masculinity in, 75; and coronavirus pandemic, 152; relations with Egypt, 6, 11, 12; September 11th attacks, 11–12; and Spanish Flu pandemic, 165n9
United States Development Initiative (USDI), 102, 109, 112, 122; funding for, 116, 121; and IVGP, 100–101, 106–7, 113–15, 123
urfi marriage, 30
USAID, 95, 130

village girls, 7, 10, 13–14, 30; attitudes regarding IVGP, 117–21; compassion for, 93–94, 95–96, 100, 101; in global aid policy, 93–94, 97, 99–101, 152, 153, 154; and *I am Nujood, Age 10 and Divorced*, 94–96, 97, 98. *See also* International Village Girl Project (IVGP)

Wark, McKenzie: on humanitarian images, 74; on images of children, 163
West Bank, 17
Winegar, Jessica: on culture, 171n9
World Bank, 6, 13

Yemen, 11, 17, 94–95, 122, 161; child marriage in, 94, 95, 98, 100

Zambia, 171n23

Stanford Studies in Middle Eastern
and Islamic Societies and Cultures

Joel Beinin and Laleh Khalili, editors

EDITORIAL BOARD
Asef Bayat, Marilyn Booth, Laurie Brand, Timothy Mitchell,
Jillian Schwedler, Rebecca L. Stein, Max Weiss

The Politics of Art: Dissent and Cultural Diplomacy in Lebanon, Palestine, and Jordan 2021
HANAN TOUKAN

Screen Shots: State Violence on Camera in Israel and Palestine 2021
REBECCA L. STEIN

The Paranoid Style in American Diplomacy: Oil and Arab Nationalism in Iraq 2021
BRANDON WOLFE-HUNNICUTT

Dear Palestine: A Social History of the 1948 War 2021
SHAY HAZKANI

A Critical Political Economy of the Middle East and North Africa 2021
JOEL BEININ, BASSAM HADDAD, AND SHERENE SEIKALY, EDITORS

Archive Wars: The Politics of History in Saudi Arabia 2020
ROSIE BSHEER

Showpiece: The Building of Dubai   2020
  TODD REISZ

Archive Wars: The Politics of History in Saudi Arabia   2020
  ROSIE BSHEER

The Optimist: A Social Biography of Tawfiq Zayyad   2020
  TAMIR SOREK

Graveyard of Clerics: Everyday Activism in Saudi Arabia   2020
  PASCAL MENORET

Cleft Capitalism: The Social Origins of Failed Market Making in Egypt   2020
  AMR ADLY

The Universal Enemy: Jihad, Empire, and the Challenge of Solidarity   2019
  DARRYL LI

Waste Siege: The Life of Infrastructure in Palestine   2019
  SOPHIA STAMATOPOULOU-ROBBINS

Heritage and the Cultural Struggle for Palestine   2019
  CHIARA DE CESARI

Iran Reframed: Anxieties of Power in the Islamic Republic   2019
  NARGES BAJOGHLI

Banking on the State: The Financial Foundations of Lebanon   2019
  HICHAM SAFIEDDINE

Familiar Futures: Time, Selfhood, and Sovereignty in Iraq   2019
  SARA PURSLEY

Hamas Contained: The Rise and Pacification of Palestinian Resistance   2018
  TAREQ BACONI

Hotels and Highways: The Construction of Modernization Theory in Cold War Turkey   2018
  BEGÜM ADALET